Reader Response

"Thank you for your precious book! Every word seems spoken from my heart—my deepest feelings, longings, fears, faith, confidence, praise... At the moment the valley is still dark, but I'm not alone."—Ann

"I am nearing the end of my treatment regime and look to the future with revived energy from having read your book."—Dorothy

"I see the depths of feeling and I can identify with all... Thank you for sharing."—Pastor Ed

"Your book is beautiful, heart-wrenching, comforting, assuring. I will come back to it again and again."—Holda

"I can understand why so many patients at the cancer clinic are so inspired and comforted by your book."—Dot (oncology nurse)

"Thank you for such an affirming and uplifting book. It is now in our lending library and I will confidently recommend it."—Riverview Cancer Care (USA)

"Your story gives me hope and courage."—Sr. Charlotte

"I was frequently overwhelmed by the freshness and rawness of your prose. I can easily understand how this book has been so meaningful to those who read it. I plan to bring it to a lady I have to visit. I'm sure it will be more therapeutic than anything I have to offer."—Henry (MD)

"Your honesty and directness are incredibly moving. It is a great gift you share."—Nandy

"What a comfort it is! I am so eager to share it with other patients and will bring it to oncology on Monday."—Phyllis

"It was as if you were in my head giving me words for the feelings I could not express."—Shirley

"Last night I opened your book and couldn't put it down. What an encouragement to hurting hearts. I've walked alongside those who bravely face this monster."—Esther

"Love of the One who sustains us during the unthinkable flows from every page. The Lord used your thoughts to awaken new springs in my dry heart."—Marg

"Your book will inspire many people and give them the will to battle the dreaded disease. Sunday is my fifth year anniversary and we're having a party!"—Debbie (The Lady Behind the Counter.)

"I hope my Mom will be well enough to read your book. I couldn't put it down. It helped me to see it all from the patient's point of view."—Chrissie (teenager)

"Your book touched me in places I didn't know existed. Thank you for writing it. Thank you for your honesty and openness. Thank you for sharing God's faithfulness."—Jean

"I could not put the book down and even when tears obscured the words sometimes, I had to finish it. I had to get to the end, I had to know that you came through it unharmed and whole. I had to find the hope. We don't know what the future will bring. What we do know is that His Hands are stretched over our family with love and protection."—Jeannetta

Tenth Anniversary Expanded Edition

The Valley of Cancer

A Journey of Comfort and Hope

Also by this author:

Seven Angels for Seven Days

Tenth Anniversary Expanded Edition

The Valley of Cancer

A Journey of Comfort and Hope

Angelina Fast-Vlaar

Angelina Fast-Vlaar

THE VALLEY OF CANCER
A Journey of Comfort and Hope
Tenth Anniversary Expanded Edition

Copyright © 2008, Angelina Fast-Vlaar

ISBN-10: 1-897373-41-4
ISBN-13: 978-1-897373-41-5

(First printed in 1999, Essence Publ. ISBN: 1-55306-022-9)

Charcoal sketches: George Langbroek
www.artsniagara.com
Mountain painting: Bruce Fast
www.brucefast.freeservers.com

For additional information please contact the author:

Phone: 905-938-1175
E-mail: fastvlaar@becon.org
Internet: www.angelinafastvlaar.com
www.thevalleyofcancer.com

WORD ALIVE PRESS

Published by Word Alive Press,
131 Cordite Road, Winnipeg, MB R3W 1S1
www.wordalivepress.ca

*This Tenth Anniversary Edition
is lovingly dedicated to
all the courageous ones
walking
through a valley.*

Contents

Contents

Acknowledgements

Thank you family, friends and colleagues, for your encouragement and assistance ten years ago to publish a book based on my own experience with cancer, a book designed to give hope and comfort to cancer patients.

Thank you, Joe, as you led this team of supporters by your constant love and patience.

Thank you to all who now encouraged me to expand the volume by adding "reflections—ten years later."

Thank you, Word Alive Press staff, for your expertise in publishing this edition as an expression of gratitude for ten added years of life.

Introduction

In July of 1997, our lives suddenly changed as I was diagnosed with colon cancer. My husband, Joe, and I were confronted with the fact that the unbelievable—"which always happens to somebody else"—was now, indeed, happening to us. Life's path took an abrupt turn and led us into a valley.

We had travelled through valleys before, having both previously lost a mate by death. What we learned in those previous difficult times came to mind again, namely: the best way to travel through a valley is to keep our hearts open to God, the Shepherd and Overseer of our souls.

Like many others, I like to keep a journal. Writing helps me to deal with the difficult things, to work through my feelings, to make sense out of life and God's work in my life. My journal this past year took on the form of a more or less poetic narrative as words and phrases came to me that spoke the feelings and carried the meaning of what I was going through. Often, as I wrote, a message emerged—a bit of Scripture tucked away in memory, a song, something I had read or was reading at the time—a message, I believe, given now to encourage me, to help me through another day.

Family members and friends have encouraged me to publish some of what I have written in order to make it available to others struggling with cancer or illness. I have arranged the writing according to the 17 months of my journey. For each month I have briefly related some of the events that happened during that month followed by some of the writing I did at the time.

A quatrain from a poem (author unknown) quoted in *Streams in the Desert* states:

If you have gone a little way ahead of me, call back–
'Twill cheer my heart and help my feet along the stony track;
And if, perchance, Faith's light is dim, because the oil is low,
Your call will guide my lagging course as wearily I go.

During our journey through the valley, there were many others, gone ahead, who "called back" to us, encouraging us, cheering us on. It is my prayer that this sharing of my journey may be a means of "calling back" to you to encourage you, whatever your valley may hold.

July

S tep by step we descend into the valley, a deep valley, and it will take at least a year to travel through it. I am glad it comes a step at a time. I see it as God's gentleness, giving us time to catch our breath, to absorb and adjust to each piece of new information. It starts with the passing of blood in my stool on the morning of Canada Day. When it occurs again, my doctor advises me to go to Emergency. I am admitted and spend a week in hospital undergoing tests: X-rays, ultrasound, blood work and the unpleasant colonoscopy. I go home for two days and am re-admitted to another hospital for surgery to remove the tumour and do a resection of the bowel. The anxious wait for the biopsy results, more distressing news and the introduction to oncology follow.

In the part of St. Catharines known as Port Dalhousie, we live close to Twelve Mile Creek. The path of this creek and its valley become a symbol to me of the spiritual and emotional valley we are travelling through.

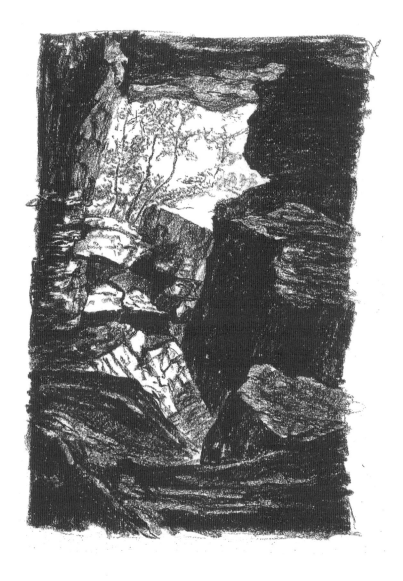

July 1

Yesterday,
I read that all the days
ordained for me
are written in His book.
Today,
I have a sickening
sensation inside.
Tomorrow,
I will see my doctor.
Yesterday,
today,
tomorrow,
God remains the same!

Hurtled into the Valley

After a week of tests
and tubes and toilets
my doctor stands at the foot
of my hospital bed
and says in an everyday voice,
"The tumour is malignant."
He pats my covered leg and says,
"You'll be all right."
His words are lost in the reeling room
that screams at me from all sick sides—
"It's cancer! It's cancer!"
My limbs freeze but
I make them move
and drag them down the hall,
repeating to myself
to make the truth sink in,
"I have cancer—I now have cancer."
I grope for the telephone.
Shaking fingers fumble to find
the buttons to press.
The ringing starts and stops
and his soft voice says, "Hello."
I'm dumbstruck,
realizing that one word
will shatter his joy,
his recent-found joy.
Finally, while choking,
"Hon, it's malignant."
A muffled groan wells up
from the depths of his loving heart.

"Oh no, my love—I'll be right there."
He comes and we collapse
in each other's arms and cling
as we're hurtled,
    crying,
into the valley of the shadow of cancer.

Later,
when our tears are dried,
we see the Shepherd
with outstretched Hands
to comfort and to guide.

He knew we were coming.

Why?

There's a shower stall
at the end of the hall
and I walk its length,
skirting the labelled doors
behind which super-bugs are raging.
    Crazy place—
    all I need yet is a virus.
I find the stall,
rip the curtain shut
and turn the faucets on—
    full blast.
Hot water pounds my face
while my sobs pound out:
    Why Lord?
    Why?
    Why me?
    Why now?

To What End?

There is no answer
*   to my "Why?"*
God need not explain Himself
and is He the author of disease?

I need to change the question
*   and rather ask,*
"To what end?"
"What will happen
if I surrender
this whole matter
into God's hands?"

Now—
I can expectantly look
*   for answers.*

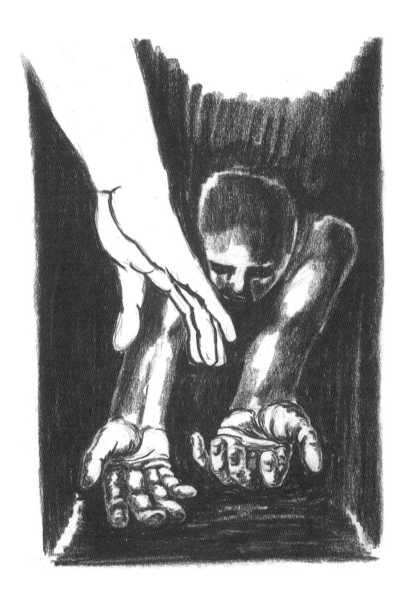

The Tumour

Malignant, damaging,
breaking the rules
by which the body
is designed to live.
Growing in seclusion,
in darkness, until its
menacing presence is felt.

A malignant, damaging attitude,
growing in secrecy
behind the closed doors of my heart,
breaking the rules
by which the Body
is designed to live.

I bring this cancer
of body and soul;
I surrender it all
to be made whole.

The First of Many Miracles

The surgeon comes to meet me. I size her up. I'm impressed. She grabs a piece of paper towel and I watch her pencil trace the curve of my colon, encircle the tumour, and with three sharp strokes capture the cursed thing within a triangle, denoting the swath of tissue to be removed.

Yes, please, get it all.

She tells me I'll have to wait three weeks for surgery. I'm shocked.

Three whole weeks? Don't you know this thing is killing me?

Her eyes meet mine. Something passes between us. She excuses herself and returns to tell me surgery is scheduled in two days.

Thank You, thank You, Lord!

The Day Before Surgery

A group of friends arrive
this Sunday morning
to worship on our deck.
We share and thank
and pray for grace
to bear what lies ahead.

Now in the quiet of this afternoon
I'm drawn to dwell on love—
the love of God.
A love so grand
I cannot understand
   how long
   how wide
   how high
   how deep
it really is and not a thing
in heaven or on earth
can separate me from it—
not even an operating room.
I see the room before my eyes,
cold metallic grey, scrubbed to shine.
But then it changes and behold,
I see it bathed in gold—
aglow with a warm Presence.
With this Presence there,
what have I to fear?

Afternoon Vision

Heaven has occupied my thoughts of late
as I am moving closer to the time
of entering, sick or not.
It's all a shiny golden scene
and a sense of peace pervades.
I close my eyes and, startled,
I see before me, faint and far,
my loved one past, immersed in light,
smiling, beckoning me
to join him in the glory.
Transfixed, I stare upon the scene
and finally turn away,
only to see my present love
beckoning me to stay.
I'm overcome with puzzlement—
is there for me a choice?
Can the balances be tipped
this way or that?
I think of Paul, who said,
   What shall I choose?
   I do not know!
   I'm torn between the two.
   I desire to depart
   yet to stay is better for you,
   for your progress
   and joy in the faith.
I look deep within my heart
and if in some mysterious way
I have a say,
I choose to stay and I pray
that it will be for joy.

Evening Prayers

It's been a busy, blessed day
with children and good friends
all wishing us well
for tomorrow.
I turn in early
but there's a knock on my door
and three little children settle on my bed.
With their father tall
their prayers are said.
Hands over my belly
they all pray for health
and I praise God
for the wealth
of love coming our way.

Surgery—Going In

I hear my name called on the intercom.
I ride down halls, around a corner—
    to the doors.
A quick kiss,
another promise to pray
and I glide into the "golden" Presence.
To think of it this way
calms my thumping heart.

Coming Out

A dark-haired nurse—
dark eyes—
a clock—
my body shaking—
hot blankets—
breathe deeply, Angie—
Joe's voice—
pain—
faces—
surrounded by love—
relief—
sleep.

The Day After

I open my eyes and see my daughter curled up in the easy chair. She smiles.

"Hi, Mom."

Every time I open my heavy eyes she's there, smiling. She reads to me as long ago I read to her, and when the nurse enters they together pamper me.

At night my daughter returns, alarmed at my exhaustion due to too much company.

She closes the curtain.

She shuts the door.

She turns off the light.

She perches herself on the edge of the bed and, while gently stroking me, she softly sings,

"The Lord bless you and keep you,

the Lord make His face to shine upon you

and give you peace,

and give you peace."

She kisses me goodnight, slips out of the room and leaves whispered instructions with the nurse at the door.

And I, like Mary, store up in my heart the treasured moments I am finding in this valley.

A Further Step

My surgeon folds herself into the chair as if relieved
to rest her feet.
The results are in.
The tumour was not contained.
It has spread to surrounding lymph nodes
and the doctor of oncology will see me shortly.

Joe throws up his hands in a give-up gesture.
   "I've lost one wife to cancer,
   God forbid that I lose two!"
The oncologist comes and gives us the facts.
   "You have stage 3 colon cancer.
   A year of weekly chemotherapy increases
   your chances of survival by 30%.
   We'll start with a five-day intense treatment,
   then once a week for a whole year.
   I'll see you in four weeks."

We're left alone
to grapple with this further step
   deeper into the valley,
a step we prayed we would not have to take.
Joe has been here before and for him
it is a dark, remembered reality—
a long gloomy corridor of pain.
I'm a mess of tangled thoughts.
We hold each other close.

When Joe goes home
I listen to the tape he left for me
and the room fills with
the beautiful harmony of,
　"Come unto Me
　if you're weak and laden,
　if you're weak and laden
　I will give you rest."

I lie back on my pillow and with "tears in my ears"
I open my heart to the love in this song—
　God's healing does not
　depend on statistics.
Somehow, somewhere, it will be all right.

Treasures

I'm in isolation, for fear of a bug.
Everyone who enters
must wear a mask and gown
and gloves and slippers over shoes.
There's a knock, and a little one
enters dressed in yellow garb
hitched up at the waist,
a duck-bill mask covering
most of her little face,
and her hands, outstretched,
have droopy plastic fingers.
She shuffles in, fingers flapping,
and with her eyes locked on mine
she says,
> *"Grandma, I love you so much*
> *and Grandma,*
> *I want you to get better*
> *and Mommy told me*
> *I could pray with you."*
It's a puzzle how to fold the floppy fingers
and a secret smile plays at her lips
> *behind the mask.*
Then, serious, she says her little prayer.
With a kiss and a hug I express my thanks
> *and she shuffles out.*
Five times the scene is repeated
with variation according to child.
And as my "treasures" leave,
I store up more treasured moments.

My Nurse from Dublin

There once was a nurse from Dublin
who loved to dress like a goblin.
All in yellow, she would say,
"Visitors, go away!"
God bless my nurse from Dublin.

There once was a nurse from Dublin
who knew not the likes of muddlin'.
She deftly could bathe,
powder, bed made!
God bless my nurse from Dublin.

There once was a nurse from Dublin;
never was there such a goodlin'.
She feared not "the bug,"
she deserves a big hug.
God bless my nurse from Dublin!

The Creek Valley

I have a hospital room with a view.
It overlooks a valley,
the valley of Twelve Mile Creek.
The banks are steep and covered
with the thick lush foliage of summer
and only further on do I get a glimpse
of the silvery sliver of water making its
way through the greenery towards a bridge.

There's a path down in the valley
winding its way along the water's edge;
Joe and I have walked this path.
It is shaded and secluded and still,
and we have been refreshed by the solitude.
Wild flowers and berries grow here
and exuberant bird song is all around.
But there is a place along this path
that is dangerous and scary—
the place where the swift-flowing water
rages as it tumbles and thunders
through a narrow rocky passage.

Toward its mouth the creek bed widens,
filling the valley with a peaceful,
shimmering expanse of water,
sliced by the slim, sleek craft of rowers
racing to the finish in summer fun.

The very end of the valley is a festive place
with shops and music and ice cream
and sand castles on the soft stretch of beach.

July

The creek is now confined within the walls
of an old canal and it bobs pleasure craft
up and down to the ancient cranked-out tunes
of a merry-go-round.
Finally, meekly, the creek is escorted out
by two long piers and is lost in a Great Lake.

In the evening, from my hospital window,
I see the sun set over the valley;
the tops of the trees iridescent now
with the amber light of the sinking sun.
But further down, the valley's sunless sides
are black with eerie shadows
cast on the dark ribbon of water
snaking its way below.
It looks menacing, this deep night valley.
I would not relish being there alone.

The sun slips out of sight.
I lower the blind with a sigh
and climb into bed.
What will my valley of cancer
hold for me this year?
Quiet solitude?
Leisure time?
The dangers of a lonely darkness?
The agonies of a narrow place?
But maybe—
there will be a wider place,
a peace—
a losing of the drop of myself
in God's "Great Lake" of Love.

The Lady Behind the Counter

We find the little shop that sells drug-free meat and free-range eggs. Joe calls me over to meet the lady behind the counter.

Her dark brown eyes are filled with love as she says,

"I had cancer and I am well. I was bald and now look at my hair!"

Her fingers comb her long dark tresses as Joe's hand strokes my shoulder. He senses the importance of this first meeting with a survivor in the community of which I now am part.

I hesitate to share—(do we tell the size of our tumours? The length of our scars?)

"My cancer is stage three," I softly say.

"Mine was stage four," she simply says and smiles.

She is one who has gone ahead and is calling back now to encourage me. I sense my step grows a little lighter.

The following week we return, and as she waits on us she asks, "What is your name? We've been praying for you all week."

August

I have four weeks to recuperate from surgery. It's a bittersweet time. We rejoice that the tumour is gone, yet there is a realistic apprehension at what may lie ahead. I take time to read about the subject that now so occupies our minds.

There seem to be so many pieces to the puzzle as to why a cancerous tumour may develop. The literature speaks of genetics, stress, a weakened immune system, cell mutations, pollution, harmful chemicals in processed food, diet. Authors speak of the close connection between body and mind as a "seamless web." Our mind, emotions and spiritual well-being all influence the physical body, and as they may have played a part in allowing cancer to develop, they can now play a part in beating the disease.

There is no doubt in my mind that I need to follow the conventional chemotherapy treatment route, but I decide to brew Essiac tea, make carrot juice, take some supplements and make an appointment with a naturopath.

I buy *Chicken Soup for the Surviving Soul*—stories of numerous battles fought and won with cancer. I sense a host of people calling back to me: Have faith, have hope, fight! Have courage to take the treatments; follow the cancer-fighting diet; saturate yourself with the positive; pray and surrender all to Him who "heals all our diseases."

Chemotherapy treatments begin in the middle of the month. I receive intravenously 700ml of a drug called 5-Fluoride. This will strip my gastro-intestinal tract, killing the faster-multiplying weaker cells, which hopefully includes any cancer cells. (It also includes skin, nail and hair follicle cells.) Levamisol, an immune booster, is prescribed to be taken over a three-day period every other week. I am told the Levamisol tablets may give me flu-like symptoms but the 5-Fluoride is unlikely to make me ill and seldom do patients lose their hair. I am encouraged.

The treatments start with a dose every day for five days. When I report a tiny blister in my mouth after the first dose, the nurses look at each other and say, "We have someone here who is going to react differently." After five daily treatments, all hell breaks loose.

A Wasted Year?

Some say that this will be
a wasted year.
That depends on the measure.
A work-quota yardstick
may find it wanting
but the lessons
learned in solitude
may be beyond measure.

Help Along the Way

Bundles of books
Amazing articles
Timely advice
If it looks promising, I'll view it!
Healing herbs
Cleansing teas
Veggies and fruit
Beta carotene
The whole diet regime, I'll do it!
Prayer and faith
Support and love
Visualisation
Relaxation
A positive spirit
All this will get me through it!

Child/Stepchild

I see fear in your eyes—
*   you have lost a parent and it is*
*   unthinkable*
*   that death should strike again.*
I see courage in your eyes—
*   a determination to pitch in*
*   and help us bear this burden.*
I see maturity in your eyes—
*   you are acquainted with valleys*
*   and have travelled through your own.*
I see hope in your eyes—
*   all cancer is not fatal;*
*   there are new treatments,*
*   new alternatives.*
I see faith in your eyes—
*   you know where our strength lies;*
*   you know the God who answers prayer.*
I see love in your eyes—
*   you unabashedly draw near and*
*   surround us with it and we feel it*
*   like a protective hedge.*

Grandchildren

You bring us joy and lift us up.
We see your unpretentious
curiosity, faith and love,
and you remind us to strive
to become more like you.

First Visit to Oncology

*"Today is the day," we courageously say, and drive
to the Hotel Dieu Hospital.*

Elevator, second floor.

"You've been here before," I venture to say.

*"I know every square inch of this place," he replies,
with a bite in his voice.*

*"Two rounds, two years apart, only to lose her in
the end."*

*The nurse is kind and gives him extra time to deal
with the* déjà vu.

*We walk down the halls to the brightly painted walls
of the remodelled "Chemotherapy Suite."*

*We leave, our minds spinning with all the
instructions, my body feeling the effects of destruction,
and our hearts aching for all the sick people we saw.*

Emergency

I wake at 5 a.m. and pace the floor.
My mouth and throat are now
completely bubbled with blisters;
my bottom lip is one long thin balloon.
To take a sip of water
feels like gravel going down.
I pace and sob and vent my angered
anguish at this ordeal.
Emergency, Oncology says.
Gentleness surrounds me here.
IV—no swallowing required,
Demerol, to ease the pain.
A private little curtained space,
a box of tissue all my own.
I turn my face to the wall and
suddenly remember
King Hezekiah did the same.
He wept bitterly and prayed
and the Lord saw his tears
and heard his prayer
and gave him fifteen more years.

Relativity

All things are relative
   they say.
The pain in my throat,
   my mouth,
is only relative to the pain
   of my cancer.
If this attack on my mouth is any
indication of how aggressively
the cancer cells are being attacked
   in my colon,
then I "gladly" bear the pain.

Swish and Swallow

"Swish and Spit" and "Swish and Swallow" are the nicknames for my two medications; the first to prevent, the second to freeze the blisters in my mouth.

I stuff the Swallow in my purse as we leave for an outing to Albert's on the water. Before the meal arrives I steal a private moment in the ladies room.

Rats!—forgot the spoon!

*I place the bottle to my lips and take a swig—*anyone looking to start a rumour?—*then swish and slowly swallow the thick red stuff.*

Back at the table my numbed-out taste buds try to remember the exquisite flavour of the creamy shrimp-filled crepes before me on my plate.

The Lion King

The little lion lies low in his den
while we courageously deal with
the telltale signs of his presence.
    Pain—
    Distress—
    Loss of an organ—
    Loss of a limb—
We hold the beast at bay
(for years and years sometimes)
until one day
he roars out of his cave
    pounces—
and the obituary reads,
"After a courageous battle with cancer..."

However—
one of the elders said to John:
    Do not weep!
    See!
    The Lion of Judah
    has triumphed!
    He is able!
    He who sits on the throne
    spreads His tent over them.
    He leads them to springs
    of living water.
    He wipes away every tear—
    To Him be praise
    and honour and glory
    forever!

September

I get nearly a four-week break to recover from the intense five-day treatment. Then the once-a-week treatment routine starts and I am assigned to have mine every Thursday.

I plan to keep my life going as near to normal as I can and activities are scheduled for the beginning of the week with my group work at a local school on Wednesdays, my best day.

I tack jokes and quotes on the fridge. A favourite is, "All the necessary supplies have already been provided for this journey." I make it a point to laugh—it's an immune booster.

We are out for breakfast on the last day of August and I absentmindedly run my fingers through my hair and pull them back—full of hair—no laughing matter! I spend this month dealing with all the various aspects of going bald.

A friend is going through chemotherapy also and I write the Glory poem for her. I treasure all the cards we receive. The messages in them often are just the very thing I need for that day. I am humbled to know that so many are around us, thinking of us, praying for us, and this gives me a sense of being carried. I also treasure the little angel gifts I receive: a bear, beautifully crafted pins, angel cards—they are reminders of the gentle spirits' promised presence.

September

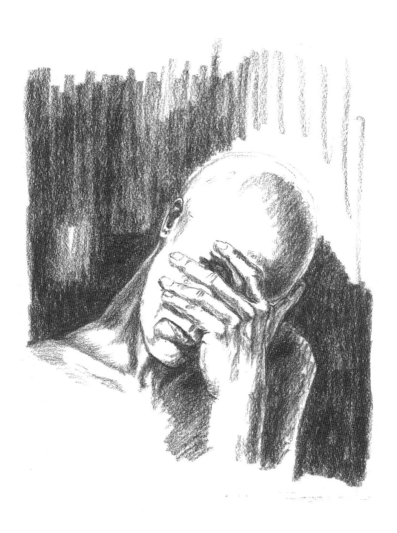

Losing It

It's the burial day of Princess Di
and, therefore, a good time to cry
about the hair I'm losing.
I know there's no comparison
but it's a treasured part of me
and I feel diminished.
So, as I watch the mourners on TV
I run my fingers through my hair
and mourn each fistful that my scalp
lets go. I place it safely in a bag—
*   after all—*
you can't just put it in the trash!

Hats

Today—hat shopping with my daughter! The last time we went shopping for a hat was for her wedding and that was quite a while ago.

I try on the creations, prance around, leave hair behind in each and quickly pluck it out—dear me! I'm glad we've talked about the loss; today we can laugh as we try to discover the art of fashioning a hat.

"I could easily make this for you, Mom," she says, dipping her voice to a whisper. "I'll just measure with my hand."

I choose a classy burgundy felt and we go for tea.

Back home, I spend the evening searching out the many scarves I, in my pack-rat mode, have saved throughout the years. I try to wind and twirl and tie the cloth around my balding head and model them for Joe. I find some woollen knits to keep my chilled head warm, especially at night, and I am glad another step is taken.

Memories of Courage

My hair is thinning fast and I phone Joshua for advice. My 13-year-old grandson replies,
"Just get the vacuum cleaner out!"

I remember the Sunday afternoon nine years ago when all his hair came out at once. His younger brother got the vacuum to swoosh away the hair and in a fit of laughter placed the hose on Josh's head—a moment of comic relief in the staggering struggle.

I remember the shock of leukemia, the burden of weekly chemo for two long years. I remember the brave little boy with "Mr. Hickman" in his chest. I remember his prayers, his favourite hat, his smile, and I say to myself,
"If he could do it, so can I."

Glory—for Jane

My glory is slowly vanishing!
First a fist full, then a brush full,
a sink full, a whole bag full!
Appalled, I look in the mirror.
My hair, my glory, given me as a
covering is getting unhinged
and with horror I watch it go.
A hairless creature stares back
at me, eyes brimming with tears.
Surely that is not I!
The tears spill—we cry—
Finally, gingerly, I reach out
and embrace what now is me.

Jesus said that every hair of my head
is numbered and that not one
shall perish without His knowing.
I ponder these words and hear Him say,
    Draw close, my child;
    let My love be your covering.
    Feel My hands
    upon your hairless head
    and hear My tender words
    of compassion and comfort.
    Rest, relax, I will cover you
    during this time of trial and tears.
    And when your beautiful hair
    has all grown back there will be
    glory of a deep dimension
    because you have walked with Me.

The Wigs

We drop in at the
Cancer Society Office
where they graciously offer
    for free
a wig or two or three!
So what will it be?
Red ringlets?
Raven black hair?
A mass of brown curls?
Or something fair?
We laugh and giggle
as I change my looks
and pick out two
that fit the books.
Then to the little ones
to share our find.
They are overjoyed
that I'd be so kind
to let them be the models.
After all the jolly good fun
I gather my hair
from reluctant fingers
and take it home to be laundered,
treasuring the memory that lingers.

Look Good, Feel Better

Tonight, Jane and I attend
"Look Good, Feel Better."
We're taught about
skin care and hair care
and where the eyebrows should go
and dots to fake our lashes.
Then come the hats and scarves
and we're shown some clever ways
to adorn our hairless heads.
We share our stories and one by one
we gather courage to remove our wigs
and reveal our various states of baldness.
Empathy and encouragement flow
especially to the one still facing the fact.
Then, with our wigs replaced
and faces made up,
we do look good
and we do feel better
and express our thanks
for this timely help with our disaster.

Of Hats and Hair and All Things Fair

What shall I wear?
My hair or my hat?
A big decision like that
requires careful consideration!
So
I try on my hair
I try on my hat
I try a bright scarf
and decide with certain elation
to wear all three.
So
I plop on my hair
I plop on my hat
I tie the bright scarf
and stand back to see my creation!
Such choices I have
with a hairless head
I can give in
to my crazy, wild imagination!
My "covering" is gone
but I am all right
for Love covers me still
and to Him goes my heart's adoration!

My Journey

Lord, the path looks so steep today.
It looks downright treacherous
and tomorrow I have to continue the climb.
It's a year's climb—and I'm afraid.
I fear what lies ahead.
How much poison can my body take?
What damage will there be?
Will there be healing?

> *My child,*
> *I know the way that you take.*
> *It's a difficult route*
> *but this is the way*
> *for you to travel this year.*
> *You know My presence*
> *goes with you.*
> *I am always near*
> *to comfort and guide.*
> *Learn of Me.*
> *Lean on Me.*
> *Lean hard.*
> *Leave your care with Me,*
> *for I care for you—*
> *deeply.*

Pathway to Healing

The ten lepers must have felt foolish
walking to Jerusalem all covered with sores.
The blind man must have felt ridiculous,
eyelids caked with mud, groping
to find his way to the pool.
Naaman must have felt humiliated,
accustomed to carved marble baths
filled with sparkling water, now riding
to the Jordan to dunk himself
seven times in a muddy river.
And how do I feel sitting on a recliner
while a nurse pushes a plunger
to fill my veins with poison?
I feel sick and bald.
Yet, this is my particular path toward
healing. So, like the others,
I will trust and not be afraid.
I will think of the chemo as Hope.
I will pray and eat well
and take my pills
and thank the Lord for the
peace that comes as I,
believing,
set out on my pathway to healing

October

I t bowls me over how ill I get after each treatment and I wonder how in the world I am going to last for a year. I stick my nose out the back door during "pill week" and tell Joe there is something wrong with the pond. The air smells putrid. The coffee odour in the lobby at the hospital is overwhelming and I ask the nurses if they've had a chemical spill as I gag at a whiff of the clinic. They remind me that the Levamisole has heightened my sense of smell. I find it disconcerting to think that the sweet smell of earth, especially after rain, may in reality be not that sweet at all. I'm glad this new affliction will be with me only a few days every other week.

My naturopath is a lifeline, literally. She has time to listen and knows of the routines and ravages of chemo. She opens her cupboards and selects for me the help I need. Amazing! My blood count goes up, my energy increases, my bowels settle down and I get a better night's sleep.

My tattered old copy of *Streams in the Desert* becomes my daily companion again. The Psalms take on new meaning. I read that, "Nothing under His control can ever be out of control." (*Intimacy with the Almighty*, by Charles R. Swindoll) I want to keep my mind and heart open to God's love and wisdom and strength.

Split-Week Personality

For three days
*   I lounge around in my robe*
*   moaning "sick"*
*   with no energy nor*
*   interest to do anything*
*   except to sleep by the fire*
*   or hole up in my room*
*   deep under the covers*
*   fighting this major "flu."*
Then there is a day of transition
*   and for the rest of the week*
*   I'm up and dressed,*
*   trying to sing a happy tune,*
*   delving into projects*
*   with gusto galore*
*   which instantly evaporates*
with the next visit to oncology.

Black Thursday

Days of feeling well
enjoying life and all its joys
are abruptly ended by the coming
*   of Thursday.*
A few pills, a needle pulsing
poison through my veins
are enough to collapse the wellness
and I am catapulted into a world
where the air smells foul,
where the water reeks,
where food and drink take on
a strange metallic taste,
where my stomach revolts,
my mouth breaks out,
and my muscles turn to lead.
I curl up by the fire on the soft
*   sheepskin rug.*
How sick can I get? Will I
bounce back before next Thursday
already looming black on the horizon?
The glowing fire warms my shivering
frame and I remember reading,
*   "May the Lord direct your*
*   hearts into God's love and*
*   Christ's perseverance."*
As my body relaxes in the fire's
warmth, I let my heart relax
in the warmth of God's love
and I muse how Christ's long
dark Friday turned to "Good"

because He persevered
to work a great salvation. But
how can I persevere through
a whole year of Thursdays
coiled before me like
an ever-circling, menacing maze?
And so I cry,
   O Lord, direct my heart
   that I may learn to persevere
   through all the "good" Thursdays
   and may they work towards the end
   that I'll be free
   from this dreadful "C"
   D.V.

Autumn Praise

Winding down a crimson-coloured
　country road
　　a child bursts forth in song.
　　　In clear high notes
　　she sings her self-made psalm
　circling around
the colour of the leaves
　the beauty of the fall
　　and praise to God
　　　who made it all.
A hush descends as we're swept along
　for miles of worship
　　seeing through innocent eyes
　　　the golden leaves become the
　　streets of gold, so smooth
　so perfect for her roller blades!
As her song winds down
　another voice begins
　　rising and falling
　　　until her song crescendos
　　in high notes of praise
　which slowly descend and end.
The holy hush lingers and prompts
　a prayer to rise and take on words:
　　If this should be my last day here
　　　may my farewell
　　be filled with praise
　spontaneous and sincere
as the praise that You ordained
　from children's lips sung here.

November

I read about the power of the mind and the power of faith in the healing of our bodies and I determine that if my weeks are reduced to a few days, I will try to concentrate on the positives in those days. A cartoon now on the fridge reads, "Yesterday's the past, tomorrow's the future, but today is a GIFT. That's why it's called the present." I try to weave the "thread of gratitude" into the fabric of my daily life and look for "haunts of happiness."

A little poem by Mary Butts (quoted in *Streams in the Desert*), which I memorized years ago in another valley, comes to mind again:

Build a little fence of trust around today;
Fill the space with loving work and therein stay.
Look not through the sheltering bars upon tomorrow;
God will help you bear what comes of joy or sorrow.

It somehow helps to visualize my day as protectively hemmed in. It reminds me of the hedge that God put around Job; nothing can touch us without God's permission.

The drug has a cumulative effect and by the middle of the month I fail to bounce back and am still ill when I arrive for my next treatment—too ill to have any more. My doctor tells me to go home and try to get well and says that he will reduce the dosage by 50ml.

It's distressing to discover I have an adverse reaction to the better anti-nausea drugs and I have to settle for Gravol and Zantac and try to make the best of it.

Day and Night

Thank you, Lord, for four great days filled
with gold and crimson and purple and blue.
Days filled with love and warmth and joy.
Days of peace and praise.
Days filled with children's laughter hiking
on a sandy shore, squealing in a windy shower
of rain and golden leaves whirling all around
like so many blessings strewn upon my path.

Tomorrow at 11:00 a.m.
I will be leaving this world of joy and fun,
descending again to a place of distress,
holed up in my room deep under my covers
battling the baffling chemo.
But in the depths of darkness seeds germinate
take root and sprout and they will blossom
when sun and light arrive
on my next few days of wellness.

The Treatment

I'm nauseous before I get to my appointment. It's all in my head—anticipatory.

The needle prick is a jab again. The drug starts to seep in and I feel my whole body revolting at this intrusion. It's as if all my cells are crying out,

"No, no, we are whole. We don't deserve to be destroyed! Why should we have to be wiped out just because a few deformed demons are hiding somewhere?"

The nurse is kind. She gives me another Gravol and phones in yet another prescription for the unrelenting nausea.

Joe holds me close as we walk back through the cold to our van. On the bridge over the Creek, near where the water rages, the drug strikes full force, knocks the wind out of me and I sink into my seat with a long low groan.

Home—Please hurry—Home.

A Slippery Path

I feel as if I'm walking on a
     slippery path
just never knowing when
it will be dry enough to take
a further step or will it get so wet
that I'll fall flat on my face?

"When I said, 'My foot is slipping,'
Your love, O Lord, supported me."

Face-Off

The "C" monster seems large of late.
And mouthy.
He taunts,
> *So you're getting sicker, I hear.*
> *Any "well" days lately?*
> *Are you beginning to catch on to who I am?*
> *I take and take until there's nothing left to*
> *take. And I can outsmart the chemo,*
> *you know. I go into hiding. Just a few of*
> *my cells, that's all it takes, and at the right*
> *moment we start the onslaught again.*

After days of cowering behind fears and
tears I finally face the foe.
> *Well, big mouth, you may think you can*
> *take and take but you have to wait for*
> *permission to be granted!*
> *Besides, your taking is so limited.*
> *You can't take away the diamonds I saw*
> *sparkling on the fresh snow this morning.*
> *You can't erase the love received in a card*
> *the mailman brought.*
> *You can't undo one word of the special*
> *sharing with a daughter nor delete, "I love*
> *you, Mom" on my e-mail messages today.*
> *You can't wipe away the love washed all*
> *over a little child's face as she slips her*
> *arms around my neck and whispers,*
> *"I'm so glad you're here."*

Never can you drive a wedge in the love-
bond I share with my husband, let alone
do anything that would separate me
from the love of God.
You see, you can't touch my spirit, nor the
things of the spirit, and healing lies in the
power of the Spirit.
So, big mouth,
you may brag about imagined strength but
you are a slain foe and total destruction
awaits you sooner or later.
Life and love and complete wholeness
lie in store for me now and forever.

End of battle—for now.

"Haunts of Happiness"

"Haunts of happiness"—the nooks and
crannies in my life where little joys abide,
sometimes hidden by a veil
when I ran here, then there.

Orange blobs, motionless now in the pond,
slowly sinking lower, totally surrendered
to the darkness that lies ahead.

The stately maple's long bare arms
reaching to protect our house.

A squirrel squeezing into the round
door of the birdhouse on the fence,
exiting with a look of triumph.

My room—drenched in vanilla
in the morning light.

My books, old friends, lined up along
the wall, still speaking long after
I have shut their covers.

Lacy patterns projected on the wall
by the late-afternoon sun.

Rhythmic dancing in the hearth.

The whispered bursting of bubbles
around me in my bubble bath.

The way my husband's eyes hold
a smile before it reaches his lips.

"Varied and rather unaccountable"
are these spatters of joy.

I'm blessed to live in a place where
my spirit feels at home,
a place filled with many
"haunts of happiness."

December

The highlight this month is that my hair is starting to grow in. The five-day treatments destroyed the hair follicles but the weekly drug dosage is not enough to continue the destruction. The reduced dosage of the chemo drug helps to give me a few good days each week again.

It's a struggle to realize I will not have energy to do the usual Christmas preparations and celebrations. The children, of course, pitch in and treat us this year to dinner in their homes. I learn that the true meaning and blessing of Christmas remains, no matter what the external circumstances may be. A poem written nine years ago brings comfort now.

The Dance

My tiny daughter was
    placed in my arms
        and I danced.
She had soft dark hair
    which I caressed
        to the steps of the dance.
I brought her home
    and we danced
        through the house
            in the garden
                on the street
following the
    Lord of the Dance.
We whirled and twirled
    and circled about
        moving close and far
            and closer again.
She placed her first tiny
    daughter in my arms
        and we danced.
She had velvety soft hair and
    I stroked her head
        to the steps of the dance.
We danced to the beat of her music
    inside and out
        on swing on sand and sea
our steps in mysterious harmony.

This grandchild cuddles close
    and we dance tonight.

With my wig removed
  her strong young fingers
    dance on my bald head—
      a massage to help
        my hair to grow.
She squeals out her surprise:
  "Grandma, there's new hair
    growing all over your head!
      It's very, very soft!"
My daughter joins and deftly
  cuts old straggly strands
    and tenderly shapes my
      quarter-inch hair.
"It's so soft, Mom!
  It's dark and white
    and maybe curly too!"

This dance tonight
  is a wondrous thing.
We whirl and twirl and
  come full circle.
For now my head
  with newborn fuzz
    is loved and admired
      as theirs once was.

Grace in the Dark

It's a dark day today.
So many dear ones
and no energy to attend.
I am shutting out
the ones who love,
the one who loves me most.

It's a sad day today.
The things I enjoy so much,
working, sharing, shopping
are too much just now,
and I am shut off
from the excitement of life.

It's a troubling day today.
The eight months before me stretch
like an unending path
of being shut in.
What happens to relationships
if they become a one-way street?

It's a thoughtful day today.
A day to open the Living Word.
"My grace is sufficient for you."
"In quietness and confidence
shall be your strength."
"I am the Lord who heals."

It's a prayerful day today.
A day to open my heart to the Lord.
Give my loved ones sustenance,
give us strength
and help us all to draw from
Your well of unending grace.

Advent

Mary could not make
lavish preparations
to receive her Son.
She simply opened her heart.
With all the tinsel stripped away
the Gift becomes the greater.

Christmas Giving

Mary giving herself
to be the mother of God,
bearing stigma and shame.
Joseph giving himself
to be father to the Child
he had not fathered.
The innkeeper giving
a stable and clean straw
and didn't his wife come
running with a bowl of broth?
The angels giving a
rousing rendition of their
Hallelujah Chorus.
The shepherds giving
adoration in the middle
of the night.
The wise men giving
their costly gifts and
worship to a tiny Baby.
God giving His Son—
the greatest Gift of all.

A Little Child
(December, 1989)

*She snuggles into my arms
finding the perfect fit.
Her small hand reaches to touch my face
and contented crooning escapes her lips.
Her big brown eyes slowly close
and her tiny body relaxes
totally trusting its weight to my care.
She sleeps.
I stand in the soft glow
of one electric Christmas candle
and contemplate the depth of my love
for this beautiful granddaughter of mine.
If I, in my finite sinful humanness
can love this little child,
can I not believe how much
my heavenly Father loves me,
His child,
and can I not completely relax
in His loving everlasting arms,
entrusting my total being to Him
and become as a little child?*

January

A new year. What will it hold? I feel so much that we are in the dead of winter in more ways than one and in this sense it will be a long winter. I realize that, despite the many sick days ahead of me, which I am definitely not looking forward to, this coming year is a gift of time to let my body heal, to let my mind be taught, even to let my spirit soar?

I find it distressing to see new people at the clinic continually—the bald heads, the wigs, the pallid skin, the fearful stare—but there is also laughter and so much bravery and constant words of encouragement from accompanying family. My appreciation for the staff who work so cheerfully among us rises increasingly. "Dot" mentioned in "Angels on the Battlefront" is a play on a nurse's name.

I figure out the best time to come to the clinic to avoid the long waiting line; I bring my own heat pad to save the time it takes to get some vein nice and plump in my winter-cold hands. My treatment lasts only as long as it takes to inject 1300ml of liquid into a vein (half drug, half saline solution). Some patients have to wait for hours, a day, or overnight for the bags of drugs to empty.

Joe brings cheer to the clinic. He jokes with the nurses, chats with the patients, listens to them, has an encouraging word. He holds my hand, avidly studies my blood work chart each week and gets tears in his eyes when a vein pops. He is not a doctor but everyone is blessed by his excellent "bedside manner." He tops my daily gratitude list.

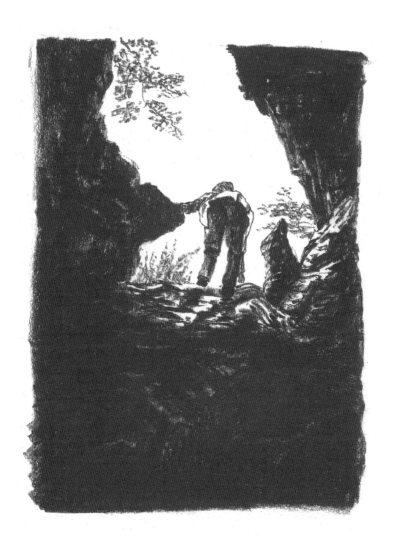

January 1

A new year,
mercifully
behind closed doors
which open only enough
to let a moment slip in.
I used to stand on tiptoes
waiting to see
what they would bring.
Strange, that today,
in the midst of all this uncertainty,
I have a sure sense that I know
exactly what many a
long-drawn-out moment
will hold.

Yet,
"Moment by moment—
I'm kept in His love."

Cold!

I awaken to another Thursday
and look out the window
    to see it snow.
Why is it always raining
    or snowing
    or blowing
on Thursdays?
Nature's empathy?
I shiver just thinking
about how the cold hits
me after the treatments
as we make our way
to the van. I crawl back
under the warm duvet.
Joe comes to check
on me and I say
that there is no way
    I can go today.
He lets me be—
brings me tea—
With a look of deep
concern he says that
    I must go.
Go for myself and
    go for him.

With a prayer on my lips
I go once more.

Warmth!

*I am humbled by
the love we are receiving.
It so encourages me
to keep on believing.
It wraps itself
around me like soft fur,
keeping me warm
during this icy winter.*

The Pits

Is there a pit in this valley?
I seem to have fallen into it
    and cancer is all around.
One buried, one dying, two diagnosed,
one being operated on today.
We're in this pit together, I guess,
    all trying to climb out.
Some make progress but then fall back.
Some just give up.
Some courageously, painfully,
    climb to the top
and are granted a few more years
or so it all seems from this pitiful stance.
Where do I fit in?
What will my outcome be?
"I called on Your name, O Lord,
    from the depths of the pit.
You heard my plea…You came near
and You said, 'Do not fear.'"
I thank You that
"My times are in your hands"
and that You
redeem my life "from the pit."

Angels on the Battlefront

I enter a den of bulging bottle bellies,
trailing plastic tube tentacles—

> *"Would you like a bed or a recliner?"*

lurking to latch on to me.

> *"Something to drink? Juice?*

A stench wafts up my nose—

> *"Here's a scented candle."*

and makes my stomach turn

> *"Do you need a bowl to vomit in?"*

as I'm led to my chair of execution.

> *"I'll just stroke your hand awhile."*

A tiny tendril fastens to my vein—

> *"Sorry, did that hurt?"*

lethal liquid seeps into my blood

> *"Some ice in your mouth will help."*

in search of cells to be destroyed.

> *"Here's an afghan to keep you warm."*

The battle rages.

> *"You're doing well. I like your hat."*

Gentle beings Dot this den—
float here, then there—

> *"Shall I turn the music up?"*
>
> *"Would you like to watch TV?"*

ministering spirits—

> *"Is there anything I can get for you?"*

making the battle bearable.

> *"Shall I close the door?"*
>
> *"Draw the curtains shut?"*
>
> *"Tell me about your children."*

The Companion's Valley

I wonder if this illness
isn't as hard
  or harder
  on Joe
than it is on me.
Sure, I am the one who struggles
  with the chemo
  week by week,
but he has to watch it all
and often the frustration of
not being able to make it better
grates on his tender soul.
The fun times are also gone for him;
the lonely times increased; the
burden of household duties multiplied.
He journeys through a valley
  all his own
as he so caringly and lovingly
walks by my side through
this winter of our lives.

February

We are reaching the halfway mark. It's a time to rejoice that we've come this far, but I am very aware of how far we still have to go. My oncologist is sensing that it's becoming too big a struggle and he suggests I skip one treatment to give us a holiday to build up some stamina for the rest of the year. Two weeks of sun in Florida, squeezed between tornadoes and storms, shines like a blessing upon us. As the quiet days pass, some energy returns and somewhere deep inside, God-given for sure, we tap into the courage to continue treatments.

Dear Lord

I thank You for the chemo
even though tears are so close
to the surface.
I thank You that there is a chemical
that can kill most cancers
if they have not advanced too far.
I thank You that
in the grand scheme of things
    You are in control,
healing this body by whatever means
    You choose.
Help me to be in step with the healing.

Blue Eyes

His eyes are what catch your attention
in the weather-worn face
softened by snow-white hair
still thick and soft.
The vivid sky-blue of his eyes
is so clear and intense
that invariably you gaze
a little longer than is warranted.
That is how I responded the first
time his eyes met mine—
*   before he was mine*
and thus I have seen others respond.
I've seen a little child's gaze riveted
and adults finally letting go
with a sigh exclaiming,
"His eyes are so blue!"
But colour is only a partial description.
These blue windows draw your gaze
into a soul that is large and full of love.
It's the love that makes the blue sparkle
*   as sun shining on a sea.*
It's love that softens the blue
as he speaks that empathetic word.
It's love that bathes the blue in liquid
as he remembers pain
or feels the pain of someone else.
He is one of God's blue-eyed creatures
graced with the gift of love.

Pillow Talk

"Despite this constant
feeling ill,
somewhere deep inside
I feel so well,
so healed,"
I whisper,
cuddling close.
"I know."
"What do you mean,
'you know'?"
"I just know deep
in my heart
that you're healed,
that you'll be well."
"How do you know?"
"I think God told me so."

March

This seems to be a month of reflection as I read and reread some favourite authors. I ponder how families react when lives are changed due to illness.

I adjust to the rhythm of my days, each day defined as to where I am in this roller-coaster ride, and I find that familiarity brings with it a certain amount of stability.

I am reminded again of Gibran's words in *The Prophet,* "The deeper sorrow carves into your being, the more joy you are able to contain."

And someone says to me, "It came to pass, it did not come to stay."

Prayer

My prayers are snatches of thought—
    a word here,
    a thank-You there,
    a sigh—
I'm glad my Father loves me
and understands I am too
    tired to pray
    today.

At night,
Joe comes to pray with me.

Refiner's Fire

Placed in a crucible
over a flame
my song-less soul
gives way
gives up
the impurities clinging within.
The Master skims the surfacing dross
and watches and waits
for His image to appear
glimmering on this mess
of sinful humanness.
It is enough.
He lowers the flame.
The song returns.
Refined.

Tested and Tried

I visited Marble Beach
on Australia's eastern shore.
Hemmed in by massive rock cliffs
it holds a rich store
of perfectly polished
smooth, round stones
and I selected some
to take back home.
I watched the succession of
waves in their continuous roar
come up and rattle and clatter
the stones on the shore.
They are rolled and rubbed
against rock and sand
relentlessly, ceaselessly
ground by Nature's fair hand.

Sometimes I feel like a stone
on that faraway beach
as God's ways leave me in
anguish and I beseech
Him to stop the pain and the
grief that comes o'er and o'er.
Yet, He knows the path I tread
and what lies in store.
Job said, "When He has tested me
I will come forth as gold."
"A polished arrow," I became,
said Isaiah of old.

I do not know the plans
God has for me in His grace
but I must trust His hand
in the challenges I face.

Transformation
(After reading Kay Arthur)

Our disappointments are His appointments.
Change the "d" to "H" and leave a space
for often it takes some time
before we see the "good" of His working,
conforming us more and more
into the likeness of His Son.

Family Ties

The family's the place
where connections are made
determining
personhood
identity
safety
stability
how the family fares
when the storms of life assail
when challenging changes come
for come they may.

The family where
members are connected
by thin threads of
surface formalities
trivialities
dishonesties
rigidities
totters precariously
and like a house of cards
collapses with the slightest
gust of change.

The family where
members are connected
by strong cords of
unconditional love
sincerity
honesty
elasticity
stays intact, whole
and like a fortress strong
can survive the fiercest
storm of change.

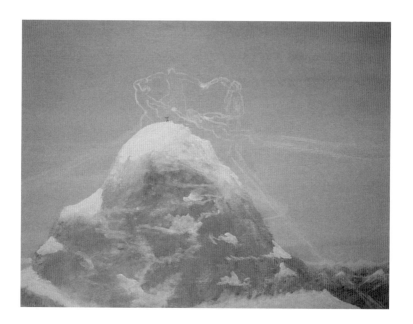

The Mountain Top

I receive one of my son's paintings—a scene of a grey-white mountain range under a vivid blue sky with one snow-draped peak rising above the others. On this peak are three translucent figures—dancing—while assisting a fourth to join. Vapour trails, like those that airplanes leave behind, sweep around the mountain depicting each figure's course of ascent.

It is dedicated to me.

I seem to hear strains of "Love lifts us up where we belong," floating from the canvas. Also, the rush of eagles' wings as the figures soar, exuberantly joyful as they "ride on the heights of the land."

I express my thanks in a note and say that mostly I struggle in the climb but sometimes I soar!

The Kingdom of Love
(After reading Hannah Hurnard)

Kingdom children are filled with love, for love is the rule of the Kingdom.

Kingdom children are filled with holy desire which their Father, the King, places in their hearts.

Kingdom children perform holy wonder—the miracles that happen when hearts full of love, spurred on by holy desire, reach out to those in need.

This way the King is magnified.

This way the Kingdom spreads.

April

Spring is in the air and with it comes the joy we experience each year as we see the garden slowly come to life again. It's always a reminder that after the death of winter comes the resurrection of spring. But this month, with another friend diagnosed with cancer, death still stands in sharp relief against the signs of resurrection.

Even though I'm convinced I will live for now, I think about death and what it will be like to die. I imagine saying good-bye—and it makes me cry. It prompts the Easter poem.

I share with a long-time friend, also struggling with cancer, that, as Christians, we just can't lose. To be granted extended years here will give us great joy; to be called Home means a still greater joy awaits us.

Good Friday

A needle slips into a vein
in my hand and it hurts.
Especially when it misses
and the nurse has to jiggle it
or pull it out and try again.
I wince with pain. But
what is that compared
to nails being hammered
through both of your hands?

I take to my bed for a few days
because the chemicals put
into my body make me ill.
But what is that compared
to your body hanging on a cross
and being left there to die?

Sometimes I can't sleep
and I pace the floor and cry
and wonder what the future may
hold. But what is that compared
to being awake all night
fully aware of the hell to come
and the agony of that being so great
that your sweat turns to blood?

Sometimes I get hurt
when someone is unkind
or when someone I love is angry.
But what is that compared
to having hundreds hate you
those in authority flog you
make sport of you
spit at you
push thorns into your head
and crucify you?

Sometimes I think
I suffer so much.
And then I think again.

Easter

I am waiting here for the angels
listening for the rush of wings
straining to hear the grand invitation,
"Come here, my child, enter in!"

There's a swishing, a swirling, a lifting
of spirit from body, bound for decay.
We fly through a tunnel of brightness,
arrive at the gate of pearly array.
It opens, I hear singing and shouting,
"Enter, you're welcome, you're Home!
We've been waiting and watching and praying
that you'd be faithful until you came."
My loved ones are lined up to greet me,
my friends, my relations and all
throng around to guide and lead me
through the golden, brightly lit hall
right to the throne of the Saviour.
A hush falls as elders bow down
along with thousands of others
each dressed in a snowy white gown.
I bow, I adore, and I worship
My Lord, My King and My Song.
I praise Him for keeping me safely,
for giving me strength to hang on.

I am waiting here for the angels.
Do I hear the rush of wings?
Do I see bright creatures approaching?
Will I now see what eternity brings?

The Sun Still Shines

The doors are locked this morning;
The blinds are tightly drawn.
A dismal dirge of mourning
Drifts across the dawn,

Spirals me down toward the grief
Locked in my heart, now quick to spill.
The floodgates open, strange relief
To let the surge go where it will.

My heart cries out, it's been so long!
So sick, so long, to lie so still.
My soul somewhere has lost its song,
My flesh too weak to spur my will.

Upon Your grace I thus am cast.
Help me, Lord, Your face to seek.
I lean upon Your promise past,
"My strength prevails when you are weak."

I see the Sun crack through the door,
I lift the blinds to let it shine.
Its warmth pervades my soul once more
And with the Light comes peace of mind.

A Rude Interruption

It's warm and sunny today.
Spring flowers are blooming here
   and at my neighbour's.
Squirrels scamper along the picket fence,
birds are busy building
and there are baby fish in the pond.
Everything around me speaks of life
but my neighbour is dying—of cancer.
Three months left to live
   on our friendly street
where we chat, visit over coffee,
laugh at each other's wit,
inspect each other's gardens,
tell how the children are doing,
know when the lights go out, when
the car is gone and when it returns.
Who wants to leave?
   I don't.
   He doesn't.
We're in the midst of life and in this
sense death seems like a very rude
interruption—the last enemy
come to snatch one away
while we're in the middle
   of the play.

Yet, when we are on the other side
   clothed in immortality,
we will fully understand the mystery:
"Death has been swallowed up in victory."

Meeting Alvin

While out for breakfast this morning,
I met a saintly man whom
    I've known for years.
The cancer in him has been held at bay
but now a fiercer onslaught has begun
    which many of us would fear.
I placed my hand upon his shoulder
    and looked into his eyes.
They glistened with a tear as he
said with a smile,
    "I've served my Saviour long-
    distance for ever so many years,
    soon I'll serve Him in His
    very presence and it will make
    it all worthwhile."
His face shone with a certain glow
as he was speaking of the end
which is for him—
    the beginning.

May

ay turns out to be my most difficult month. I am sick continually, I am an emotional mess and there is something within me that says, "Enough! This is all my system can take." It makes me think of the narrow place in the creek valley where the water spurts and sprays against the rocks.

My oncologist explains that my body has reached saturation point and if the immune booster pills make me ill, it only means that they are working. The nurses remind me again of the detrimental effects of the chemo on my emotional well-being and the social worker encourages me to be gentle with myself.

The oncologist strongly recommends I continue with the treatments and says, "We're not talking about feeling ill this summer, we're talking about being well ten years from now." He suggests I skip one treatment to give myself a much-needed break and "then we'll talk again."

Weeping

Three months left of it.
I'm so sick of it
and tears course down my face.
Someone has said of it,
"It's the body weeping
for what has been done to it."

The Roller Coaster Ride

*Up and down
and round and round
this roller coaster speeds.
The tracks are set
and twist and turn
and roll relentlessly.
I've had enough
of high to low
can someone stop this monster?
I need to get off!
Let me escape!
I've had enough already!*

*You can't! You can't!
Get off and—what?
Stay on, stay on!
You're right on track.
Go with the roll—
surrender to what is!
Doze through the downs,
ride on the highs—
the wind blows through new hair!
Stay on, stay on!
You must stay on
your ride to health again!*

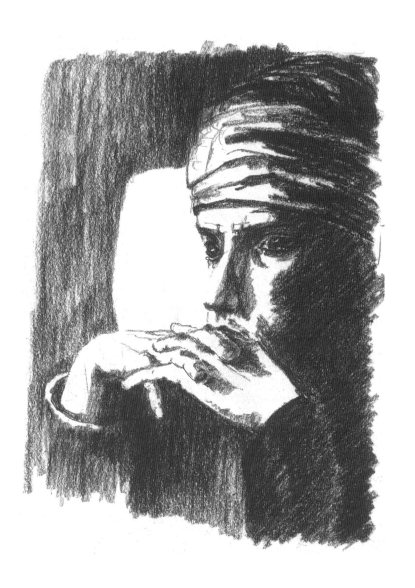

Time Out

I escape into the van—
park it by the lonely beach.
With blackened windows it's
my private thinking chamber
where tears can flow at will.
Eight months of illness is taking its toll.
I feel so disconnected, stranded, alone.
Everyone has gone ahead while I linger
behind, struggling to get through this crazy
year of scheduled illness.
There was a fork in the road
as in Robert Frost's two roads
diverging in a wood. Others stayed
to the right but I was directed to take the left
and plod "the one less travelled by,"
following a different beat of the drum.
It sounds like a dirge.
Others speak of solitary journeys:
a sculptor releasing a figure from stone,
a writer following characters on a page,
a painter stroking, stippling, dabbing, led
along by an inner guide.
I need to consider this. Something
is being fashioned, written, accomplished.
I know not what but
*   "He knows the way that I take,"*
and that is enough for now. I must
bravely journey on toward the "sun-rising"
when all will be brought to light.

This Old House

My nails are now so thin
they curl over my fingertips,
*   hawk-like,*
if I let them grow.
The tissue-paper skin on my
hands stretches over veins
distended and discoloured.
My mouth is blistery again
my nose bleeds
my ears get jabs of pain
my stomach is distressed
and what is the condition
of my innards by now?
"My harp is tuned to mourning
and my flute to the sound of wailing."
But while I wail about this wasting,
a flash of truth suddenly clears
my horizon:
*   "...we do not lose heart*
*   though outwardly we are*
*   wasting away, yet inwardly*
*   we are being renewed*
*   day by day."*

Comfort

A comforter—
someone who comes alongside,
who can bear to be with me,
to walk with me,
and for a moment sense
the contours of this path.
The Comforter incarnate.

Cross

My looking well
is deceiving and
things   are   ex-
pected of me which I cannot
fulfill—on time. Some do not
understand my limitations and
have been cross.
But then—do I
really understand
someone   else's
c   r   o   s   s ?

"Come unto Me"

I play the cassette tape Joe brought to the hospital over and over. The song "Come unto Me and I will give you rest," touches a deep cord of longing within.

"Take my yoke upon you and learn of me," Jesus said.

I visualize a double yoke like one I saw in my uncle's old barn. Jesus walks with me. Or, rather, I walk with Him. That's why He says, "My burden is light."

The Double Yoke

My **LORD** says to **me**
My yoke   is easy
My burden   is light.
He invites   me
to ease   myself
into the   part of
His double   yoke
designed   for me
and walk   in step
with Him;   my burden
now is light because
He   carries
the   brunt
of   it.

Narrow Places

The jagged
rocky
sides
of the valley
are pressing in on me
and I cry out in
anguish.
I sputter and tears spatter
as I stumble
through this
narrow
place.
It all has to do with
being housebound
continually ill
missing out
and feeling unable to
take yet another treatment;
family members
ailing
aging
moving
and the list goes on.
My backpack is stuffed
to ɔ full!
It's toɩ difficult
to travel this
narrow
path

with all
of life's burdens
on my back.
It's best to travel light
and leave
my cares with
Him
who cares for me.
My pack deflates
and there is room to move
ahead.

Oncology Angels

"You can wait in the Quiet Room,"
the nurse gently says
after my doctor's appointment.
It's small and pleasant
perfectly private for
    talking—
    crying—
    praying—
    being still.
I sit on the comfortable sofa
and glance at the framed photo
of a lady, my age, whose passing
brought about this room.
The social worker settles herself
in the matching green chair
and offers her time. Together
we explore the hurdles I am
experiencing and the kaleidoscope
of emotions that whirl around
like a spinning top. An hour
flies by and, still weepy,
I leave for my treatment.
A volunteer spots me
and offers a soothing
cup of hot tea.
The treatment nurse is gentle.
Her eyes convey
empathy and care.

When finished,
I leave—
my body ill,
my heart deeply grateful
for the many who brighten
and lighten this day.

Quiet Room Wisdom

"If you put yourself at the bottom of your 'pile' how do
you expect to have energy to heal?"

***

"'No' is a complete sentence. It needs no explanation.
You simply need to learn to say it."

Wake-Up Call

My cancer speaks to me:
Wake up!
Your body is mortal
and in need of repair.
Your heart is the centre
and its beat is out of step.
Too much pounding is wasted
on the importance of "I,"
on what people are saying,
on a relationship gone awry.
On work piling up,
on what will happen next,
on unanswered questions
and what's in the future for me?
Let your heart learn to trust
and let its beat be in step
with the Father's.
Then your body will have
energy to heal,
to repair
that which was damaged
in your wake-up call.

June

I accept my doctor's advice to take the treatments to the very end and a certain amount of peace comes from that acceptance. Joe and I make some plans to help me get through another ten weeks. We decide to buy a roll-out awning to cover our south-facing back deck, so that I can enjoy the out-of-doors and be shaded from the sun and even protected from the rain. Joe plants quantities of flowers to beautify our yard and encourages me to let my body rest. We arrange for my treatments to be done on Tuesdays instead of Thursdays so that I may enjoy more of a weekend. At the clinic I can have a bed in a private space for my treatments and that works better for me than sitting in a row of recliners.

I struggle to come to terms with the fact that I will be ill most of this summer also and I continue the challenging task to focus on just one day at a time. I listen to a tape of dear friends singing this song for me a decade ago:

"One day at a time, dear Jesus,
That's all I'm asking from You...
Lord, help me today, show me the way,
One day at a time."

As the greenery and flowers grow all around me I realize that there are still many "haunts of happiness" for me to search out and enjoy this summer. I am reminded that the most important thing is not what is happening to me, but rather my reaction to it. I have a choice every day regarding the attitude I will embrace for that day.

Good News

Finally the results are in of the latest test. My score is well within the normal range, meaning that, as far as this blood test is concerned, there is no active cancer within.

"It's only an indication," they stress, but we are full of thanks.

Strange, how the valley looks wider, the sun seems brighter, our hearts are lighter—and when did all the birds begin to sing?

New Hair!

I now have a mop of dark and white curls—(also called grey).

It's really quite hilarious! The balding men in our family are more than somewhat envious! What they have lost has not grown back, yet I get all this hair! And what went on inside my skull to make the colour change? And who, at this late date, gave me my Grandma's curls?

I just run my fingers through it all and say, "Thank You, Lord!"

A Vigil

Our living room windows
wink at each other
past porches, lawns and flower beds
and the quiet tree-lined street
that runs between our houses.
Behind our neighbours' window,
hidden by the bounteous Blaze
of roses climbing up their porch,
a vigil is being kept.
We see the children come
and go continuously, silently,
as they try to say farewell
to their dear father.
Behind our window we
keep our own vigil of sorts;
our minds preoccupied—
sending up a prayer for
peace in his passing,
shedding a tear
and grappling with the
gravity of this disease
which also has me in its grip.

Sunday morning early
before dawn
he left to enter his
"Sabbath rest."

Peace

"I have stilled and quieted my soul"
after the turmoil of the narrow place
and I am ready to settle for solitude
and gain the blessings therein.
I'm content now to quietly lounge
on our deck that Joe has adorned with
flowers, standing, hanging, trailing,
blooming with showy colours against
the white trellis surround.
I while away these lovely summer days
listening to bird-song and waterfall
surrounded by my favourite books and music.
At twilight I light the little lanterns
hanging in the tree and candles all around,
transforming this spot into an enchanted
garden, too beautiful to leave,
so I stay and sleep outside
through the magic of the night.

The Valley of Baca

Today, I am reminded that
the pilgrims' path to Jerusalem
led through a valley.
Real or figurative, they
called it the Valley of Baca,
    meaning
a place of mourning and grief.
But it states that in their grief
they made the valley
    a place of springs.
I hear them say to me:
Dig a well in your valley!
Provide refreshment
for your body, soul and spirit
when the path is hot and dry.
Take a leisurely bath
resplendent with fragrant oils.
Read a good book in the shade.
Have tea with a best friend.
Take a walk along the water.
Most of all,
    "Take time to be holy;
    speak oft with your Lord."
This way you will be enabled
to finish your climb
one step at a time
    on to your Zion.

July

The achiever in me pushes now to persevere and I determine that I will hang in right to the very last treatment. I will get an "A" on this chemo course!

With all the busyness of summer stripped away, I learn to enjoy stillness and realize again that "in quietness and trust is your strength" (Isa. 30:15). I am drawn again to Henri Nouwen's meditations on solitude in his books *The Way of the Heart* and *Out of Solitude*. He calls solitude "the furnace of transformation." In solitude my "scaffolding"—the things that usually "prop" me up: the places to go and people to see—is gone, and I come face-to-face with who I am. It is in solitude that we discover that "being is more important than having, and that we are worth more than the results of our efforts."

We are blessed with a great number of beautiful sunny days and the garden is a constant joy. I listen to a relaxation tape that often puts me to sleep during the day outside. We go for walks along the Creek when energy allows, or drive to the beach and sit on a bench sipping a cup of tea.

Countdown has begun—the end is in sight!

Be Still and Know

I walk the short block from my home
and sit on the bank of the Creek.
The valley is wider here and its width
is filled with water glistening in the
summer sun, its wandering borders
frilled with leaf-green lace.
This lovely dark-watered lake has
been dubbed a "pond"—
    misnomer for sure.
I prefer to think of it, as surely
Anne Shirley would have, as
"The Lake of Shining Waters."

Last summer my view was from a fourth-
floor hospital window and all I could see
then was the valley's narrow scary depth.
Now at a different time,
    with a different view
I ponder the peace of this place.
It tugs at my heart.
I listen to hear it speak.
It is silent.
I tune in to the silence
and then beyond my ears my spirit hears,
"Be still, and know that I am God."

Reflections

The clinic is so quiet this morning,
so few people, no noise or unrest.
I think it's a picture of my journey—
I've come to a place of rest.
I want to reflect on my year in the valley—
to thank for the friends, faithfully there,
who understood my erratic mood swings;
thank for our families, my curly new hair;
the prayers offered, songs still singing,
visions of heaven and those gone before;
His promises never failing,
Him blessing us over and over.
We wouldn't have experienced these
treasures found on a low valley floor
had it not been for Him leading us
to this rich and bountiful store.
A store in the depth of a valley?
His ways are past finding out.
When we think all has been lost here
He comes and turns it about!

Questions

It's gone on for so long that illness and cure get confused.

"Grandma, when did you get chemo?" Meaning, when did you get this terrible disease that keeps you from seeing us?

I cup the serious little face in my hands and explain once more that the cancer is the illness and chemo the cure but it's the chemo that makes me ill.

She crinkles her nose as if to say, "That makes no sense at all."

I assure her it will soon be over, just four more weeks. She flashes a smile and with a glint in her eye she says,

"But I do like your hair better now than before!"

***

"Grandma, you will get better, yes? Because I want you to be there when I get married, and when I have babies I want you to hold them."

"Precious child, your wish is my deep desire."

Dancing, Again

The sky is such an azure blue today,
the air smells fresh and clean;
the garden's colours fairly dance
        and so do we.
This week's treatment brought
a minimum of nausea and pain
and the joy of seeing the end
        rolls me on a high again.
We must do something fun today:
a walk to the "end of the valley,"
a simple supper at a café,
a walk along the water,
a bench to sit and rest and chat
with neighbours and friends who also
enjoy this peaceful spot
        at the end of day.
We wander back through dark
and quiet streets and see a car
parked out in front.
        "Grandma, are you home?"
        "Grandma, are you sick?"
(This year's coupled phrases.)
Then shouting back to parents
and for all the neighbours to hear,
        "She's not sick! She's not sick!"
It's hugs and kisses and a reminder
of a birthday two weeks hence
        and the promised outing.

I assure them it will happen
because in two weeks I'll be
finished, done, over,
>   *complete,*
>>   *free!!!*
We wave them all good-bye and
Joe turns to me and asks,
>   *"Why was this day so full of joy?"*
A whirl of thoughts floats through my mind—
a line from Garth Brooks shines:
>   *"I could have done without the pain*
>   *but then I'd have had to miss the dancing."*

Making Port

The point of our journey
is to make port,
to arrive at our destination.
(Present and future, that is.)

The course of the valley
now filled with calm water
leads right into Port.
(Dalhousie, that is.)

I thus have this image,
this constant reminder
to keep travelling and trusting.
(With confidence, that is.)

August

Finally, the year is coming to a close. Thankfulness overflows. There is the last treatment. Joe buys flowers and I arrange them into a centrepiece and stick the "Oncology Angels" poem among them as a thank-you to the staff. The nurse-in-charge gives me the treatment and Dot pins a daffodil on my dress as my graduation diploma. Then it's hugs and thank-you's all around and we leave the Chemotherapy Suite, never to return, we pray.

A week later, my oncologist, who has become a trusted friend, checks on me one more time. He congratulates me for hanging in to the bitter end. He tells me he will give me a thorough check-up every three months during the coming year and a colonoscopy will be performed in three months' time to make sure there are no cancer cells remaining.

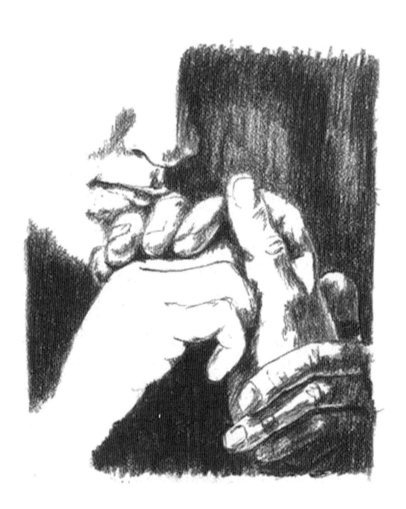

Hands

(Words of thanks to our congregation)

The time has finally come
*   to climb up and out of the valley*
and with these last few steps a deep awareness
*   rises of God's loving Hand holding us*
*   supporting us throughout this year.*
We look back and I am moved
*   as I see God's Hand made visible to us*
*   through human hands, your hands.*
We see them stretching back
*   the whole length of the valley*
*   supporting, sustaining, tending to us*
*   through all these trying months.*
First there were the doctors' skilful hands,
the nurses' gentle hands
*   holding my hands*
*   rubbing them, patting them*
*   to encourage a vein to rise.*
Then there were Joe's loving hands—
*   patiently attending, never tiring,*
*   always gentle.*
The hands of our loving children and grandchildren
*   continually caring and encouraging,*
*   giving us hugs,*
*   vacuuming our floors*
*   and keeping our mirrors polished.*
There were hands laid on me for healing.
Hands that keyed many an e-mail message.
Hands that wrote timely, encouraging words
*   on numerous notes and cards that kept*

coming and coming and coming—
that didn't stop coming throughout the year.
There were hands that crafted paintings
hands that carved a pair of hands
hands that etched hands around a balding head
and hands that painted the porch.
Hands that baked a cake, a savoury dish,
that brought us fruit and flowers and gifts.
Hands that dialled our number
that folded around our coffee mugs
for many a cheery visit.
There were little hands that printed big letters
and coloured red hearts
and drew pictures to decorate the fridge.
There were hands helping Joe when he was injured.
Hands laid on our shoulders
hands speaking love and concern
giving us a gentle push when perseverance ran so low
and hands that held us when we cried.
Still I see more hands all along our valley path
hundreds of hands, folded and lifted up
in prayer.

We are humbled.
We have been richly blessed.
We are deeply grateful
and we lift our hands up to the Lord
and reach them out to you
in heartfelt thanksgiving.

Last Treatment 1

Tomorrow is the last treatment
and strangely I dread it as much or more
than all the others gone before.
I thought I would get used to them
but that did not occur and rightly so.
I'm glad my body operates to reject
that which is foreign and harmful to it.
I pray my soul finds grace to do the same.

Last Treatment 2

It's the day after and I am sick in bed. The bell rings and I hear soft voices among a strange rustling sound. Joe gingerly opens the bedroom door and walks in with a gigantic bunch of colourful flowers in crackling clear wrapping.

The card says,

> *YIPPEE!!!! YAHOO!!!!*
>> *It's over!*

and is signed by one of Joe's children.

While my nose is in the flowers Joe tosses another card upon the bed and nonchalantly says:

"This was in the mail."

I recognize the handwriting but my "chemo-brain" can't make the connection. I open it and read a poem of tenderness and devotion. It is signed,

"I love you."

"J"

With thankful tears, I make the connection!

The End of the Valley

We're going to the beach today
We're singing and shouting hooray!
The festive place at the end of the valley
Denoting that we've finished our journey.

We've travelled a year and we've made our port
So today we'll celebrate in Port!
We'll stroll around and walk the pier
We'll enjoy the cool breezes here.

We'll listen to music and have ice cream.
We'll wander through shops; they'll see us beam.
We'll find a café that serves café au lait
And have lunch and eat all that we may!

In the evening we'll sit on the soft white sand
And watch the cool water lap the land
The sky will turn colour of every hue
And we'll thank and praise Him for seeing us through!

Stepdaughter

Who is a stepdaughter
but one removed by a step
    from being my own?
She is one who let me step into her
family, who let me walk in step with
her Dad who is so dear to me.
She who once stepped next to him
is still a precious memory
and in a sense, dear also to me.
Because she bore this daughter,
loved her, trained her, influenced her
    to be a loving soul
    who now has grace
to walk in step with someone new.
A step can be so small.
A step can be so large.
My stepdaughter has taken kind steps
this year to help me step through
my difficult valley of cancer.
She has made my step a little lighter.

Dear daughter, sister, friend,
I count it a privilege to walk
    in step with you.

September

It is truly a time of resurrection; I am ecstatic that it's finally over. However, we find our dancing and shouting strangely subdued. After my last check-up, we found ourselves outside the hospital doors in the summer sun with a strange feeling of "Now what?" We realize now that the weekly visits to the clinic have been reassuring and comforting despite the pain. The chemo each week took care of any aberrant cells trying to develop; my blood and general well-being were closely monitored—we felt cared for. Now we are on our own and there is a three-month wait to get the final results. It seems so long to wait. I remind myself how I started this journal:

Yesterday,
today,
tomorrow,
God remains the same.

The road back to normal has its own hurdles as I realize that the drugs will take a while to work out of my system. The oncology staff told me to give myself a good six months, even up to a year.

All Things New

The infernal nausea
is disappearing.
My taste buds are in tune again!
The air and water
smell clean
and with new eyes I see
our loved ones,
our beautiful home,
the garden.
It's almost like
I've been gone a year
and now have returned
to find new joy in all that
He so richly gives.

The Road to Normal

My body is adjusting to life without the powerful drugs that have been injected all year. It's been surprisingly difficult as my system seems so out of whack. I feel like I've gone "cold turkey" except I have no clue about that.

Days of tears turn into joyful laughter. Debilitating fatigue comes interspersed with spurts of energy. It's been a roller-coaster ride of highs and lows and somewhere in between my "on" button for sleep has been mislaid.

Aroma

The late September sun
shines warmly on the deck
and I bask in the lingering days
of this year's extended summer season.
The birds have congregated overhead
and carry on a heated departure debate,
their raucous chirping
almost drowning out the
soothing sound of running water.
A sweet scent wafts its way around me
and I inspect the pots of fading flowers
searching for the sender of this delight.
The air is still—
There is no breeze—
The birds have called a truce.
My eyes roam around the yard and rest
upon the blooming vine
hiding our fence with billowy clouds
of tiny star-like flowers.
"It's the vine," I murmur and
marvel that its delicate fragrance
can so fill this garden space.
As I revel in this wonder,
I cannot help but wonder about the
"aroma of Christ."
Do others sense
His sweet scent,
"the fragrance of life,"
as they pass by?

October

Such a beautiful month of warm weather and fall colours everywhere. I relish the fact that slowly more energy is returning and find it so exhilarating to be able to be involved in activities again. This year's Thanksgiving is truly a feast. "You turned my wailing into dancing…and clothed me with joy" (Ps. 30:11).

Someone remarks to me after reading this manuscript, "I guess you were so busy getting back into life again that you only had time to write one piece. Very accurate observation!

Thanksgiving

I sometimes count my years by
    Octobers.
Memories in sharp relief tucked
among the coloured leaves of each
Thanksgiving season.
    A family photo in our woods—
    A hike on nature trails—
    A child with cancer
       carried on shoulders—
    A death so far away—
    A diamond and ruby
       engagement ring!
This year's Thanksgiving
revolves around the exhilaration
of renewed energy as I bound up
and down the leaf-strewn hills
squealing with the rest of them.

November

Finally we can say that the valley has ended! We have travelled through it and made it—praise God! The colonoscopy is done on Remembrance Day. It's interesting that I started and ended my journey on a national holiday. Rightly so. For me these days will now always carry an additional special significance.

We cannot help but reflect on the fact that this year of cancer and chemotherapy has had a profound effect on our lives.

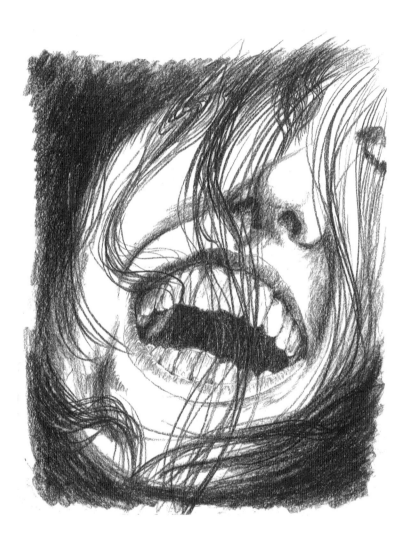

Remembrance Day

A day to be remembered
    always.
The battle's done
    and won.
The doctor's gentle voice:
"There's nothing here—
it's completely clear."
I'm wheeled out
    lying still—
jumping for joy.

Gratitude

I rub my eyes, it is so bright
in this fair land of health!
What joy there is, such peace reigns here
and all around such wealth!
I'll never be the same again
having traversed the vale.
Complacency and carelessness
were lost along the way.
A wider love now fills my heart
compassion is renewed.
How quickly now my eyes are moist
when I just hear "that" word.
In this fair land of gratefulness
each day is such a gift.
The Master reigns
and I, His child, am tripping
over my words of thanks.

In Remission

*I share the good news of my healing with someone
today and she replies,*
   "So, you're in remission."
   *The words jolt me. I believe I'm healed, but
according to the medics, I am in remission.*

   But then—aren't we all?
   *The words encourage me to keep on living a healthy
lifestyle, to keep on appreciating each day, to keep on
having a thankful heart, to keep on believing that*
      *"He will cover you with His feathers
      and under His wings you will find refuge."*

A Storm Passed

A storm passed through my life.
With gale-force wind it ripped
and tore at me,
my body, looks, my faith,
relationships, security—what all.
The wind blew fierce and
left nothing unturned.
The things most solid remained so
or more and a stronger bond
resulted with husband, children, God.
Into thin air went things
that were flighty and fluff—
not worth keeping anyway.
This cyclone sucked at the sugary dust
lodged in the crevices of "you and I"
and exposed reality.
Is there lasting fill for the hollow
or do I need to face the fact
there is no substance?

A storm passed through my life—
and left it changed.

Reflecting on a Year with Cancer

I have come to think of cancer as a big shake-up, as the "Storm" poem reflects. My attitudes towards life, my body, the food I eat and what I consider important were all more sharply focused for me this year. It's as if I were placed on a mountaintop (in a valley!) where I gained a clearer picture of my life, the preciousness of it, the fragility of it, the brevity of it, the essence of it.

My story has a happy ending. I am very aware of the fact that other stories do not have the same ending. Yet, many of you know, as Alvin did, that the final end of our stories here means a glorious new beginning.

"Every year you grow, you will find me bigger," says Aslan to Lucy in *Prince Caspian* (C. S. Lewis).

These last 17 months have also been a time of growth, and yes, I have found God "bigger" than ever before. Maybe I find Him thus because I know Him better. I know more of His love, His gentleness, His keeping me in the shelter of His wings. I know more about prayer, I am more open to the healing miracles in my life, I am more aware of my weaknesses and my precarious existence here. The spiritual world is more of a reality; heaven is closer and my loved ones dearer. I am more aware of all the people who have cancer. I am more acquainted with the ravages of the disease and the ravages of the "cure." Having been the recipient of loving care, I am more aware of how important an encouraging word is; how much it means when others care. I more fully understand how God's love comes to us and how His father heart aches for the suffering in this world.

Maybe I was led to go through this year of illness partly so that I might be humbled and see anew just how big "Aslan" is.

And now I realize I have just offered some answers to the question I asked at the beginning: "To what end?"

Reflections:
Ten Years Later

God has graciously given me ten added years of cancer-free living! It's been an exhilarating "ride." So many dreams realized, so many people I had the privilege to meet and walk with, so many opportunities to share my experiences, so many new challenges to face and so many more stories yet to tell. My first thought in the morning usually is, "Thank You, Lord!"

As I reflect on my journey with cancer and beyond, my mind turns to some foundational truths which I believe have helped to keep me safe so far and will eventually help to bring me "Home." They are: grace, prayer, living "clean," the "refiner's fire," the ministry of angels, learning to be still, keeping up hope and passing on the comfort that I have received.

Grace

The beginning of my story seems so long ago now, yet the memories are ever vivid and present, and often I still wonder how I lived through that "chemo year."

I got through because of God's grace—His favour and kindness, His "abundant provision" given us for no other reason than that He loves us and cares for us.

God's grace became evident to me almost at once. On the day before we received the diagnosis, friends from BC surprised us with a visit in the hospital. They had come to pray. The next day, after the infamous telephone call to Joe, I asked him to meet me in the common room on my floor of the hospital. It's a spacious room with conversation areas, tables and chairs, a large TV screen and usually a number of people. When I entered the room that day, I was relieved to see no one else was there. Six hours later, the only person who had entered was a nurse bringing me a supper tray. Joe and I had the afternoon to be alone, to hold each other, to cry, to talk and, finally, to pray. A gift of privacy—a gift of grace. After our prayer, Joe turned to me and said, "Whatever happens, God will be there."

I was apprehensive to go back to my ward room as I now carried a dreadful new label. (A friend told me it took her three days just to *say* the word!) How would my roommates react? When I entered the room, I was greeted rather boisterously by a cowboy standing in the middle of the room—hat, boots, jeans, denim shirt, string tie—"the whole nine yards." Grinning, he said he had been waiting for me and knew my name because it was above my bed. He was my roommate's son come from the west for a visit. Without skipping a beat, he began to tell stories of daring childhood escapades on the prairies. He kept everyone in the room, patient and visitor alike, laughing the entire evening. I recognized it as another gift of grace. It was as if God had whispered, "I know just what you need; I'll surprise you with some entertainment."

The following morning, a priest visiting the cowboy's mother came to my bed to pray with me. Then a daughter of one of the patients came and softly said, "I heard what the doctor said yesterday. I've been praying for you all week."

She tucked a small piece of paper into my hands and said, "This is the phone number of a friend who brews Essiac tea for my brother. He had colon cancer seven years ago and is well. Give this friend a call. He'll make you some."

Later that day, the surgeon came with another gift. The three-*week* wait for surgery was "miraculously" changed to only a three-*day* wait.

These first few days filled with "God moments," filled with grace, set the tone, set the course for my journey. I was convinced: God is present, God is loving, God cares.

In *Wisdom for the Way,* Charles Swindoll writes, "The most precious object of God's love is His child in the desert. If it were possible, you mean more to Him during this time than at any other time....You are His beloved student, taking his toughest courses. He loves you with an infinite amount of love." (p. 190)

Someone has said, "When in a desert place, we find God's grace in the faces of those who love and obey Him."

Throughout that year loved ones would surround me and be the carriers of God's grace to me.

Open yourself to grace, expect grace, and watch God show up!

Pray

On occasion when people ask how I battled cancer and what I'm doing to keep well, I reply: pray, purge and purify.

Prayer is most important. It is paramount that we see God as the source of our healing., In his book *Cancer and the Lord's Prayer,* Greg Anderson says that prayer "treatment" is more important than chemotherapy treatment.

Prayer is the "point of access." We open our hearts and connect with the Divine. We acknowledge God and our total dependence on Him. He is our Father; He is in control.

Prayer implies surrender. We surrender our situation to Him, invite Him into the situation and look to Him for wisdom and guidance. A cancer patient said, "Victory doesn't come when the circumstances change: rather when we see *Him* in the circumstances."

Prayer means fellowship. One of the things I treasure about the year of treatments is that I learned to fellowship with Jesus. I learned to be, more or less, in a constant state of awareness of the presence of God. My prayers were short sentences here and there. At first I thought this to be irreverent. But I didn't have the energy to pray long beautifully-worded prayers, and deep in my spirit I began to understand that what I was doing was pleasing to Him—his child running to Him at odd moments throughout the day with whatever was on her heart.

A proverb states, "A man's spirit sustains him in sickness" (18:14). Communion with God nourishes our spirit. Just as our body needs food in order to live, our spirit needs to be nourished in order to be strong. Prayer, connecting with God, is the pathway to keeping our spirit healthy. I experienced how God nourished my soul and my spirit with thoughts from his Word, a song, a verse on a card, something a friend said…He strengthened my heart, my "wellspring of life," and that facilitated the journey.

Prayer also means gratitude. The year I was on chemo I began to keep what Oprah calls a "Gratitude

Journal" and listed five things every day for which I was thankful. I've continued that practice, more or less, during this past decade. Our reality changes when we consider our cup to be half full rather than half empty. A thankful heart is a happy heart. "A cheerful heart is good medicine" (Proverbs 17:22), and we need every bit of medicine available to us!

Part of gratitude is remembering past blessings. Considering how God' grace surrounded us during past trials encourages and strengthens us for what we have to face today. Moses told the people, "Watch yourselves closely so that you do not forget the things your eyes have seen or let them slip from your heart as long as you live" (Deut. 4:11).

Count your blessings! It will change your attitude.

Purge and Purify

With God all things are possible. He answers prayer. He steps into impossible situations and works His miracles. All things are possible with Him, but what are the things that are possible for me to do? Does He work the impossible if I'm not willing to do what is possible? This thought impressed me and I felt responsible to do everything in my power to battle cancer. Jesus gave the blind man the dignity to be involved in his own healing by asking him to wash the mud off his eyes. What if he had refused? Unthinkable!

We set out on a "purging" mission. We rid our house and shed of sprays and cleaning materials that contained known toxins. Gradually we made the move to more eco-friendly products. We discovered the lawn and garden did very well without toxic chemicals. I discovered that micro-fiber cloths and water do an amazing job cleaning windows and sinks!

Next, we "purged" our pantry. Reading labels on processed foods made us aware of the harmful chemicals used as additives, preservatives and colouring agents, and we tried to avoid them. Believing that over the years toxins would have accumulated in my body, I began to drink Essiac tea, a blood and liver cleanser, to help purge my system. I still drink the tea today. I also had the mercury fillings in my teeth replaced.

I was blessed to have a good family physician, yet it was very beneficial for me to see a naturopath, to have a medically trained person with a more holistic approach to healing to support and assist me during my battle. She prescribed supplements to strengthen my immune system, to help fight the cancer, to help my upset GI track, to help with everything that presented itself. My blood count went up and I told my oncologist what help I was receiving. He simply replied, "I can't comment, but it obviously is helping, so keep it up."

My naturopath also guided me to "purify" my diet. Pure, "live" food nourishes and strengthens cells, keeps them healthy and prevents cancer development, which begins at the cell level. Our bodies are what we put into them. Gradually we chose more fresh, preferably organic, fruits and vegetables, drug-free meat (mostly chicken and fish), free-range eggs, organic yogurt, whole grains, legumes, ground flax seed, good oils, soy and nuts. Since cancer cells thrive on fat and sugar, for anything else we bought we aimed for low salt, low fat, low sugar. We eventually installed a reverse osmosis water system to give us an unlimited supply of "pure" water.

More and more research is being done to discover what connection there is between foods and cancer and between toxins and cancer. The latest findings are posted on cancer society websites.

This physical purging was one thing. Just as needful was emotional and spiritual purging. God told His people that He had led them into the desert to see what was in their hearts. Of course, He already knew; it was so they would know. Our cancer journey becomes a spiritual journey as we confront what is hiding in our hearts. A lack of forgiveness may often be one of those things.

Greg Anderson tells how his "terminal" condition turned around when he finally was able to forgive the ones who had hurt him. He writes, "With our release of forgiveness, we release God's power to accomplish his will..." (p. 59).

During the eighth month of my chemo, the social worker at the hospital helped me deal with and let go of anger and hurts I was nursing. I can point to that as the time, I believe, true healing began. The freedom I felt within was exhilarating and the treatments seemed to not affect me as severely as before. Emotional baggage is a detriment to physical well-being and it may well hinder God's work in our lives. Cancer can become an opportunity for spiritual growth if we are open to it.

So the journey itself becomes a purifying experience as we submit to the "refiner's fire." Job says, "When he has tested me, I will come forth as gold" (Job 23:10). God promises us "treasures of darkness" (Isa. 45:3), and one of these treasures may well be a purer heart.

A young mom who had a double mastectomy said to me: "It was the worst of times; it was the best of times." Her family had changed—they were kinder, more loving, more appreciative of each other and of each moment.

Paul says, "This distress has goaded you closer to God. You're more alive, more concerned, more reverent, more human, more passionate, more responsible...you've come out of this with purity of heart" (2 Cor. 7: 11 MSG).

We do not ask to go into a dark night or to experience a life-threatening illness, but it is up to us to "sift" this experience for the treasure it contains.

Angels

Angels are "ministering spirits." To "minister" means to look after the needs of others—and that's what angels do. God sends them to help us, guide us, protect us and encourage us.

One cancer patient told me she was lying in the hospital corridor waiting to go to OR to remove her cancerous tumour when a terrible fear suddenly gripped her. The next moment she saw a bright light and arms stretched around her and she heard a voice say, "I will take care of you." She relaxed and faced the surgery with a sense of peace.

Maria was already in OR when she was overcome by fear. A nurse in a white uniform came to stand beside her, held her hand and said, "Don't be afraid, Maria, I'll stay right here with you throughout the operation." When in recovery, Maria asked to speak with the nurse who wore a white uniform. Other nurses checked and told her no one had worn a white uniform that day!

We visited Joan when she was in the last stages of lung cancer. Her husband greeted us with a smile and said, "Angie, we're waiting for the angels. They're already all around the house. I can hear them!"

Joan was happy to see me and, lifting her oxygen mask, shared what was on her heart. She asked if I would read her the piece from *The Valley of Cancer* that begins with "I'm waiting here for the angels" (Easter). Her husband had already read it that morning, but would I please read it again? Teary-eyed, we tried to fathom the future glory awaiting her.

When Joe and I left their home, we had the incredible feeling that we'd been allowed to spend a few moments in heaven's vestibule where unseen angels hover.

Be Still

Last night I went for a walk to the lake. I descended the long steel staircase leading down to the water and was overwhelmed by stillness. The only sound: soft water kisses on the sand. A dusky mist hung over the winter-grey water and it was as if all of nature was whispering, "Hush." I walked along the water, found a log to sit on and soaked up the silence. After an hour or so, I went home a different person. There is tremendous power in stillness.

Learning to be still, to be at a place of rest, physically and emotionally, was a big challenge for me during my chemo journey. Usually active, somewhat hyper, running, achieving, it took me about eight months of being ill and unable to do much before I "got it." My worth is not dependent on accomplishments. My value does not lie in my health, my energy, my work. God is more interested in my "being" than my "doing." God loves me for who I am, not for what I do. My value lies in who I am in Christ. It took all of eight months before I could truthfully say with the Psalmist, "I have stilled and quieted my soul" (Psalm 131:2). And, of course, this more peaceful state of being coincided with my experience of letting go, of forgiving past hurts.

I thought once I'd learned the lesson, I would not forget it. But since that time, it seems I need to learn the lesson over and over again: "Be still and know that I am God" (Psalm 46:10).

Jesus invites: "Are you tired? Worn out?....Come to me. Get away with me and you'll recover your life. I'll show you how to take a real rest. Walk with me and work with me—watch how I do it. Learn the unforced rhythms of grace....Keep company with me and you'll learn to live freely and lightly" (Matt. 11:28 MSG).

Imagine the possibility—live freely and lightly; learn the unforced rhythms of grace! A spirit of unrest and anxiety hinders the workings of hidden spiritual forces. A quiet spirit is of great value when it comes to overcoming disease.

When "unrest" rules the day or night, I try to focus on calming passages. "In quietness and confidence is your strength" (Isa 30:15). Or, as The Message translates it, "Your strength will come from settling down in complete dependence on me." Settle down, turn off the "heat," still the inner chatter, let go and let God...

In surrender we find rest. In meditative stillness we find new perspective. Periods of deep stillness enable us to go through our day with renewed emotional strength.

The mind, body and spirit are closely interwoven. What affects one part affects the whole. On a purely physical level, rest and relaxation activate our immune systems! It has been proven that 15 minutes of deep muscle relaxation several times a week increases immune cell activity. I listened to an instructor on an audio tape to learn this kind of restful relaxation. I'd often fall asleep. Also, I'd picture my strengthened "killer" cells gobbling up the rascal cancer cells, which they actually do!

Hope

Recently I read *The Anatomy of Hope* by Dr. Jerome Groopman. During his 30-year career as a medical doctor, dealing mostly with cancer patients, he has seen the astonishing effects that hope, or the lack of it, can have on illness. He claims that true hope has proven as important as any medication he might prescribe. He tells the story of a patient who bolstered hope by reciting and meditating on Psalm 23 before, during and after each of his rigorous treatments for an incurable cancer. He lived.

Hope is "an anchor for the soul, firm and secure" (Heb. 6:19). Hope is "confident expectation" of a better future, and this expectation is anchored in God. God plans to give us hope and a future (Jer. 29:11). He promises that our valleys of trouble will become a door of hope (Hosea 2:15). Hope is being able to see in your mind's eye a better outcome. Hope is powerful in battling disease.

At the beginning of January of my "chemo year," I began to visualize August—the time treatments would be finished, no more nausea, renewed energy, enjoying activities… Whenever discouragement set in concerning the long haul still ahead, I'd pull out my "August image"—my confident expectation of a better future.

Fear and anxiety activate physiological changes in our bodies that are harmful, that depress the immune system. Hope releases endorphins that elevate our mood and reduce fear and anxiety with their harmful effects.

Hope is essential to healing!

Go Tell

It was March of "chemo year." One day after a treatment, I was curled up in front of the fireplace so ill and shivery I didn't think I'd make it through the day. After several hours (and still alive!), I reached for my Bible. It opened to the Psalms and I read, "I will not die but live, and will proclaim what the Lord has done"

(118:17). The impact of the words was like an electric current straight to my heart. These words were for me—spoken to me at this time. I would get better and I was to tell what God had done. It filled me with unspeakable joy and some trepidation. First, it meant I'd publish my story, some of the more poetic writings in my journal. And this would lead to the sharing of my experiences in all kinds of settings and to connecting with cancer patients.

But I knew the verse in Psalm 118 also meant that I needed to share another story tucked away in my journals. Another story of grace—God's grace shown to me in the Australian outback in the midst of dire circumstances. It eventually became the book, *Seven Angels for Seven Days* (2005, Castle Quay Books).

It's been a thrill to speak publicly, to share my stories with different groups of people. But to personally walk with cancer patients toward healing or toward "Home," has deeply affected and blessed me. My nearly two-year walk with Evelyn was unforgettable.

Several years ago I began to pray what is known as the "Jabez Prayer." Its four short sentences often set the tone for my day: "Bless me, Lord, increase my boundaries—my influence, may Your hand be upon me, and keep me from harm…" One day while praying on my morning walk, I sensed the Spirit say, "You can't keep asking me to increase your influence and not stop in to see how Evelyn is."

Evelyn lived three doors down from me in a small square house surrounded by a high hedge. I knew her to be 87 years old, somewhat cantankerous, wanting to be left alone and forever complaining about some neighbour or relative. I had gathered these bits of information when greeting her on my walks. I hadn't seen her during that summer, so I turned, walked up her drive and with some trepidation knocked on her door. It took a long while for her to unlock it. She invited me in and promptly began to complain about her cough and the incompetence of her doctor. I sat and listened. I did so for the next several months until one day she announced the cough had been diagnosed as lung cancer. And then it began to make sense why I was sent her way. I told her about my cancer and offered her a copy of *The Valley of Cancer.* She accepted it but said it would have to wait until she had read the four books next on her list because, she explained, "I like to do things in order."

My husband and I went south for a winter holiday, and upon our return, I noticed something different about Evelyn. She was quiet and reflective and softly said, "Very interesting book. I read it three times."

She asked to read *Seven Angels for Seven Days.* Relating to incidents in that book helped her to very gradually open a window to her soul. She began to share painful memories locked away for many decades. She told me of her disappointments, her anger at

God. She would talk and I would listen and marvel at God's grace at work in her life. She made amends with family members, she expressed sorrow for not having lived a better life, and she allowed me to pray with her now and then. One day, at the prodding of another neighbour, she opened her heart to the Lord and found forgiveness and peace.

I recorded a subsequent visit in my journal:

Ev's door is always open now.
Today she greets me with,
"That's it, no more treatments.
All those tumours—let them be."
Shocked, I say, "You're so brave."
She looks at me with a light in her eyes—
something that was not there six months ago.
"I've lived a long life. I'm ready to go."
"You've come to acceptance," I venture.
"Yes, I've accepted it." She pauses and smiles.
"I think I'll give my new leather coat to Lill.
She's been so good bringing meals and all.
You know what I did at 4 o'clock this morning?"
she continues with a twinkle in her sunken eyes.
"No, what?"
"You remember the big old bear Bob gave me?
I took it downstairs with a pair of scissors
and cut it open and took all the stuffing out
and then I cut it all to pieces."
"You did what?"
"No one is getting it. He gave it to me 50 years
ago so I decided if I'm going, so is the bear!"
We laugh. We laugh a lot lately. We laughed the

day she told me she had glued her locket shut.
"No one is going to see what's in there!"
she had giggled.
"I want to show you something," she says.
She swings her thin legs over the edge of her bed
and we wander through her little house.
We look at old faded pictures on the wall:
her parents, her deceased husband, a landscape...
I sense she's beginning to say good-bye.
She hoists herself back into bed.
"I'll stay home as long as I can."
"That's probably best for you," I say.
"Lill has offered to come in and clean, etc."
We read a page from a new devotional book.
It "happens" to be about dying and flying
Home to heaven. I hold her hands to pray.
She reaches up for a hug. I gently enfold
her frail frame in my arms and whisper,
"I'll check on you again tomorrow."
"Door's open," she smiles.
"Yes, I know."
"Good night, my dear."
"Good night."

Evelyn lived a few more months and then, very peacefully, left for "Home." And she left her "heart-print" on my life.

Someone said, "When God breaks your heart, He props open the door and from then on you have a greater sensitivity toward others who are hurting."

God comforts us in our pain and asks of us to pass this comfort on to someone else.

Be Encouraged!

My passion has become encouragement. The Lord gives us encouragement and we are to encourage each other, speak encouraging words to one another.

My favourite personal encouragement is found in Zephaniah 3:17. Trudy pointed me to this passage. I first met her as a seven-year colon cancer survivor and she became one of my lode stars. When cancer reared its ugly head again, she still encouraged me mostly by her submissive attitude. One day while visiting her, she showed me a card she had received. She read the verse on it. Then, with a light in her eyes, she softly said, "Imagine, Angie, He rejoices over me with singing. He loves me so much that He sings over me!"

I couldn't remember ever reading this passage. The Lord so delights in me that He sings over me? Trudy was fully convinced, so I went home to look up this beautiful scripture that the prophet wrote. I committed it to memory and now I retrieve this "hand full" of encouragement whenever I feel down, unloved, unsure, afraid or generally "lousy."

> *"The Lord your God is with you,*
> *He is mighty to save.*
> *He will take great delight in you,*
> *He will quiet you with his love,*
> *He will rejoice over you with singing."*

May these words also encourage you as you journey. God loves you, He is with you and He is in control. He quiets you with His love and He will fulfill His purpose for you!

Scripture passages quoted or referred to:

July	"July 1." Ps. 139:16
	"The Day Before Surgery." Eph. 3:18; Rom. 8:39
	"Afternoon Vision." Phil. 1:22-23
August	"Emergency." 2 Kings 20
	"The Lion King." Rev. 4-6
September	"Glory—for Jane." Luke 21:18
	"My Journey." 1 Pet. 5:7
	"Pathway to Healing." Luke 17:4; John 9:11; 2 Kings 5
October	"Black Thursday." 2 Thess. 3:5
	"Autumn Praise." Ps. 8:2
November	"A Slippery Path." Ps. 94:18
December	"Grace in the Dark." 2 Cor. 12:9; Isa. 30:15; Exod. 15:26
January	"The Pits." Lam. 3:55; Ps. 31:15; 103:4
March	"Refiner's Fire." Zech. 13:9
	"Tested and Tried." Job. 23:10; Isa. 49:2
	"Transformation." Rom. 8:28-29
April	"The Sun Still Shines." 2 Cor. 12:9
	"A Rude Interruption." 1 Cor. 15:54
	"The Mountain Top." Isa. 40:31; 58:14
May	"Time Out." Job 23:10
	"This Old House." Job. 30:31; 2 Cor. 4:16
	"The Double Yoke." Matt. 11:29-30
June:	"Peace." Ps. 131:2
	"The Valley of Baca." Ps. 84
Jul:y	"Be Still and Know." Ps. 46:10
September	"Aroma." 2 Cor. 2:15-16
November	"In Remission." Ps. 91:4

References

Anderson, Greg. *Cancer and the Lord's Prayer.* Des Moines, IA: Meredith Books, 2006. www.CancerRecovery.org

Canfield, Jack; Hansen, Mark Victor; Aubery, Patty; Mitchell, Nancy R.N. *Chicken Soup for the Surviving Soul.* Deerfield Beach, FL: Health Communications, Inc., 1996.

Colbert, Don, MD; Colbert, Mary. *The Seven Pillars of Health.* Lake Mary, FL: Siloam, 2007.

Cowman, Mrs. Charles E., ed. *Streams in the Desert.* Los Angeles, CA: Cowman Pub., 1955.

Fintel, William A., M.D., McDermott, Gerald R., PhD. *Cancer.* Grand Rapids, MI: Baker Books, 2004.

Groopman, Jerome, M.D. *The Anatomy of Hope.* London, UK: Simon & Schuster, 2004.

Hurnard, Hannah. *Kingdom of Love.* Wheaton, IL: Tyndale House Publishers, Inc., 1978.

Nouwen, Henri J. M. *Out of Solitude.* Notre Dame, IN: Ave Maria Press, 1974.

Salaman, Moureen Kennedy. *Nutrition: The Cancer Answer II.* Menlo Park, CA: Statford Publishing, 1996.

Swindoll, Charles R. *Wisdom for the Way.* Nashville, TN: J. Countryman, 2001.

Seven Angels for Seven Days

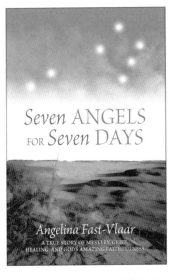

A TRUE STORY OF MYSTERY, GRIEF, HEALING AND GOD'S AMAZING FAITHFULNESS

by Angelina Fast-Vlaar

ISBN 1-894860-30-6
256 pages, softcover, $19.95
Castle Quay Books Canada, 2005
www.castlequaybooks.com

We're told that we sometimes entertain angels unaware, but never did Angelina imagine that God would bless her with, not one, but seven encounters with "angels" in the remote Australian outback.

The author and her husband are confronted with an untimely, tragic encounter while on a dream vacation in the barren outback of "the land down under." This gripping account of her personal struggle with loneliness, depression and grief is a powerful tribute to God's never-ending presence in our lives.

You'll have chills as you move from deep sorrow to the bubbling joy of God's loving presence in this amazing story. It's a faith-strengthening, must-read

Winner: "Best New Canadian Christian Author 2004"
Finalist: "The Word Guild Awards" 2006
Listed by publisher as "Canadian Best Seller" 2006
Selected by Crossing Book Club USA in 2006
Listed by Amazon.ca as # 6 Best Seller in Spirituality, Sept. 2007

Available at Christian bookstores, Chapters, Amazon, etc.